S0-AHX-827

Compression for Clinicians

Second Edition

DATE DUE
Unless Recalled Earlier

DEMCO, INC. 38-2931

COMPRESSION
FOR
CLINICIANS

Second Edition

Theodore H. Venema, Ph.D.

RECEIVED

JUN 0 9 2006

MINNESOTA STATE UNIVERSITY LIBRARY
MANKATO, MN 56002-8419

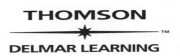

THOMSON

™

DELMAR LEARNING

Australia Brazil Canada Mexico Singapore Spain United Kingdom United States

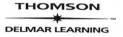

RF
300
.V46
2006

THOMSON

™

DELMAR LEARNING

Compression for Clinicians, 2nd Edition
by Theodore H. Venema

Vice President, Health Care Business Unit:
William Brottmiller

Editorial Director:
Matt Kane

Acquisitions Editor:
Kalen Conerly

Editorial Assistant:
Molly Belmont

Marketing Director:
Jennifer McAvey

Marketing Coordinator:
Chris Manion

Art and Design Coordinator:
Alex Vasilakos

Production Editor:
Kenneth McGrath

COPYRIGHT © 2006 by Thomson Delmar Learning, a part of The Thomson Corporation. Thomson, the Star logo, and Delmar Learning are trademarks used herein under license.

Printed in Canada
1 2 3 4 5 6 7 XXX 08 07 06

For more information, contact Thomson Delmar Learning, 5 Maxwell Drive, Clifton Park, NY 12065-2919
Or you can visit our Internet site at
http://www.delmarlearning.com

ALL RIGHTS RESERVED. No part of this work covered by the copyright hereon may be reproduced or used in any form or by any means—graphic, electronic, or mechanical, including photocopying, recording, taping, Web distribution or information storage and retrieval systems—without the written permission of the publisher.

For permission to use material from this text or product, contact us by
Tel (800) 730-2214
Fax (800) 730-2215
www.thomsonrights.com

Library of Congress Cataloging-in-Publication Data

Venema, Ted.
 Compression for clinicians / Theodore H. Venema.
   p. ; cm.
 Includes bibliographical references and index.
 ISBN 1-4180-0959-8
 1. Hearing aids—Fitting. 2. Compression (Audiology) 3. Hearing aids—Design and construction. I. Title.
   [DNLM: 1. Hearing Aids. 2. Cochlea—physiology. 3. Equipment Design. 4. Loudness Perception. 5. Prosthesis Fitting—methods.
 WV 274 V456c 2006]
 RF300.V46 2006
 617.8'9—dc22
2005036772

ISBN 1418009598

Notice to the Reader

Publisher does not warrant or guarantee any of the products described herein or perform any independent analysis in connection with any of the product information contained herein. Publisher does not assume, and expressly disclaims, any obligation to obtain and include information other than that provided to it by the manufacturer.

The reader is expressly warned to consider and adopt all safety precautions that might be indicated by the activities described herein and to avoid all potential hazards. By following the instructions contained herein, the reader willingly assumes all risks in connection with such instructions.

The publisher makes no representations or warranties of any kind, including but not limited to, the warranties of fitness for particular purpose or merchantability, nor are any such representations implied with respect to the material set forth herein, and the publisher takes no responsibility with respect to such material. The publisher shall not be liable for any special, consequential, or exemplary damages resulting, in whole or part, from the readers' use of, or reliance upon, this material.

6106523

DEDICATION

This book is dedicated to my two daughters, Kathryn Ashley and Angela Dawn. Kathryn came into this world on March 26, 1994 in Opelika, Alabama. She is a special child and so, her job here is not to learn, but to teach. Another angel came into our lives in Kitchener, Ontario on March 24, 1997, and so, we called her Angela. Their mother, Laura Kathryn, and I are so very proud of them both.

Contents

3 WHY SO MANY DIFFERENT HEARING AID FITTING METHODS?   42

4 COMPRESSION AND THE DSL AND NAL-NL1 FITTING METHODS   64

APPENDICES

Preface

This book is intended for those studying to become hearing health care professionals, be they Audiologists or Hearing Instrument Specialists (HIS's). It is also intended for practicing clinicians who have been out in the field for some years, and who want some refreshment of their knowledge base in hearing aids.

It is amazing how things have changed in the past 15 years. In 1990, when I left clinical audiology to pursue a doctorate in audiology, I was accustomed to fitting linear hearing aids using fitting methods based on the 1/2 gain rule. While busy at school from 1990 to 1993, the world of analog hearing aid technology had expanded considerably; for example, the K Amp™ circuits, multi-channel/programmable WDRC hearing aids, and of course, completely-in-canal hearing aids. Along with these products, new "suprathreshold" hearing aid fitting methods also began to be introduced in most of the more popular periodicals. All of these developments took place right after an exponential increase in our knowledge of the cochlea occurred in the late 1980s. The discovery of otoacoustic emissions heralded a new way of describing the role of the outer hair cells as distinct from that of the inner hair cells. This window into the otherwise inaccessible cochlea, affected the way compression was designed for those with sensorineural hearing loss. When I re-entered the real world (back in 1995), I certainly had a lot of catching up to do.

I began working at Unitron in 1995, and continued to learn so much more from them. The late 1990s were exciting days for hearing aid development. In my opinion, that time was the "golden" age of compression. Seminars in compression abounded at every conference. All hearing aids were still analog, and because of this fact, they were confined to provide one type of compression or another. Clinicians had to know these types well, because the selection of a hearing aid and its settings entirely depended on this knowledge.

The first edition of this book, published in 1998, was truly a product of my own learning process up until that time. It was an attempt to clarify and organize the many concepts that have formed the landscape of our clinical field. It was specifically meant to connect, hook, or tie together concepts about compression and hearing aids that we as clinicians had all heard before. Readers did not find new, cutting-edge research in hearing aids. I hoped, instead, to clearly explain the many buzz words relating to compression and hearing aids, and to really make them understandable to those who fit hearing aids for a living. I thought then, and still think that if this objective is met, one can apply these concepts of compression to the fitting of any hearing aid, regardless of its analog or digital origins. That's just the beginning of the story.

WHY I WROTE THIS TEXT

This is the second edition of the first book, published in 1998. Over the past 7 or 8 years, things have continued to change dramatically. Today, almost all hearing aids are digital. Basically, it had become high time to update the book if it was to remain at all relevant for today's clinicians. This book really is a bridge that spans the transition from analog to digital hearing aids. The reader will encounter many historical references. While digital hearing aids have become the norm, the complexity of their associated hardware and fitting software has also continued to increase.

The golden age of compression has passed, in my opinion, because clinicians are no longer required to understand compression in order to fit the digital hearing aids. Clinicians can simply enter the audiogram, choose a few transforms, hit some "quick fit" option, and the rest of the fitting is done automatically. Probe tube (real-ear) measures to verify what the fitting software predicts are not done as often as they should be.

Digital software has become client focused, instead of clinician focused. In and of itself, this is not a bad thing; however, fitting software has become loaded with fitting solutions that no longer specifically require much knowledge of compression. To fit today's digital hearing aids, clinicians are asked to list specific listening environments along with all kinds of psycho-social queries (e.g., does the client have trouble hearing the minister preach at a distance of 20 meters, from the left-hand side every second Sunday?).

The compression features themselves, the ones that we used to address directly, tend to be buried under the outermost layer of the fitting software. If clinicians do want to investigate what is truly going on at a deeper level, most fitting software will allow some access for further adjustments. There is, however, a real danger of becoming lost in a whoppingly complex array of adjustable features and a bramble thicket of far too many choices. Some manufacturers have anticipated this and have closed off options to curious clinicians which would compromise the sound quality their products. I suppose this is one reason why today's fitting software has taken the client-centered, listening situation inquiry approach.

It is my belief, however, that an understanding of compression in analog hearing aids certainly *helps* to understand compression in digital hearing aids. Digital hearing aids have simply incorporated various compression types and combined them together. What's more, the knowledge of compression and fitting methods, together with verification by means of real ear measures, also still applies! Just because digital fitting software has become a bit of a top-heavy juggernaut, does not mean we cannot ascertain or verify what is going on. Software simply predicts what will happen in the real ear; subsequent measurement shows whether or not the predictions do indeed take place. Far too many clinicians become mesmerized with the software, and far too few actually do follow up with verification.

Here's my final thought: To truly appreciate and understand today's digital hearing aids, one must still consult the old definitions of compression. Knowledge of compression indeed does grant more clinical power. Rather than being dazzled by all kinds of new marketing terms, clinicians can (and should) simply ask what they really mean. Armed with a healthy underpinning knowledge of compression, we can all make lots more sense when comparing and contrasting among the digital products that constantly arrive at our doorsteps.

ORGANIZATION OF THE TEXT

The book has eight chapters and two appendices. Chapter 1 provides a short description of the fascinating cochlea and highlights its hair cell functions as a "two-way street." These important additions to our cochlear knowledge base are the underlying basis of some types of compression, as discussed in later chapters. The gross function of a compression hearing aid is contrasted to the exquisite function of the active, living cochlea.

Chapter 2 describes the cochlear dead spot concept and a clinical method whereby to test for the existence of cochlear dead hair cell regions. Of course, this has huge implications for fitting methods and hearing aids; why fit a frequency region where there are no hair cells? The most fascinating thing about this concept is that in order to understand the rationale behind the test for cochlear dead hair cells regions, clinician are forced to educate themselves about the amazing physiology of the cochlea.

Chapter 3 describes a big-picture view of the field of hearing aid fitting and offers a contrast to optometry and the fitting of lenses for the eye. The vast differences between these two fields help explain why we have so many hearing aid fitting methods in the first place.

Chapter 4 offers a description of loudness growth and the necessity of compression. It also provides a short description of two popular compression-based fitting methods: DSL and NAL-NL1. In their own very different ways, these two fitting methods each address loudness growth and assume compression in hearing aids. Questions are raised about the implications of fitting with one method as opposed to another.

The heart of the book is Chapter 5, which outlines, compares, and contrasts the many types of compression available to clinicians today. Types of compression are condensed and categorized for two clinical camps of sensorineural hearing loss; mild-to-moderate and for severe-to-profound hearing losses. In this chapter, the clinical applications of the various types of compression are also described.

Chapter 6 takes things one step further and provides a short discussion on the terms "programmable" and "multi-channel" in hearing aids.

Digital hearing aids are specifically covered in Chapter 7. Various features found exclusively in digital hearing aids, including: in situ audiometry, digital architecture with respect to bands versus channels, digital combinations of compression types, automatic feedback reduction, expansion, and digital noise reduction. Some specific types of noise reduction are also discussed at length.

Chapter 8 begins with a comprehensive discussion on directional microphones and how they work. The chapter concludes with a discussion of the clinical benefits of directional microphones versus those of digital noise reduction. Despite our recent advances in hearing aid circuitry and fitting sophistication, we still have a long way to go to imitate the majesty of the human cochlea.

Appendix A is a short description of the various amplifier classes used in today's hearing aids. Appendix B contains the answers to the review questions that appear at the end of each chapter.

FEATURES

This book is quite similar in style to the first edition. One new feature to this second edition that comes to mind is the addition of review questions at the end of each chapter. Some case studies continue to be a part of this book; in this edition, these appear in Chapters 2 and 4.

NEW THIS REVISED EDITION

Much revision has taken place from the first to the second editions of this book. The topic of cochlear dead regions was not addressed at all in the first edition. This topic is now specifically and exclusively covered in Chapter 2.

Chapter 4 has also gone under extensive revision. The first edition covered four different suprathreshold fitting methods: Fig 6, IHAFF, DSL, and NAL-NL1. Since 1998, only DSL and NAL-NL1 are most commonly used. These are each given a more exclusive and comprehensive coverage in this second edition.

Also in the first edition, programmable and multi-channel hearing aids were discussed in Chapter 5, along with a scant coverage of digital hearing aids. In the present second edition, the concepts of programmability and multi-channel are discussed separately, in Chapter 6, as they relate to hearing aids per se.

Chapter 7 is dedicated exclusively to digital hearing aids. Compression as it is found in digital hearing aids, digital noise reduction, automatic feedback reduction, expansion, etc., are specifically and comprehensively discussed in this chapter.

Directional microphones were also briefly covered as a subheading in Chapter 2, in the first edition of this book. In this second edition, a discussion on directional microphones now takes up more than half of Chapter 8. Chapter 8 also contrasts the very different clinical benefits of directional microphones and digital noise reduction.

In summary, in this second edition, one chapter from the old edition has been dropped entirely (Chapter 6), and three new chapters have been added (Chapters 2, 7, and 8). What used to be a book with six chapters is now a book with eight chapters.

ACKNOWLEDGEMENTS

Just as with the first edition of this book, I want the people at Unitron Hearing to remember that I will always be grateful for the help and opportunities they gave me over the six years that I worked there. I want Paul Darkes, formerly of Unitron, then at Phonak, now back at Unitron, to know that I really appreciate all that he taught me about hearing aids. For their help and input into my very basic understanding of the various types of digital signal processing architecture, I also want to thank Steve Armstrong at Gennum, Tom Scheller of Bernafon Switzerland, and Mark Schmidt, Leonard Cornelisse, and Robert Walesa, of Unitron Hearing.

My wife, Laura Venema, took on a lot of work with our family and put up with my many absences so that I could write this book. Thank you, Laura, my love; I couldn't have done it without you. My two children, Kathryn Ashley (age 11) and Angela Dawn (age 8) continue to inspire me to be the best father I can be.

About the Author

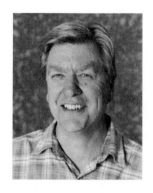

Ted Venema earned a BA in philosophy at Calvin College in 1977, and an MA in audiology at Western Washington University in 1988. After working for three years as a clinical audiologist at The Canadian Hearing Society in Toronto, he went back to school and completed a PhD in Audiology at the University of Oklahoma in 1993. He was an assistant professor at Auburn University in Alabama for the next two years. From 1995 until 2001, he worked at Unitron Hearing, where he conducted field trials on new hearing aids and gave presentations, domestically and abroad. From 2001 until 2006 he has been an assistant professor at the University of Western Ontario. He also taught part-time in the HIS program at George Brown College, in Toronto, from 1995 until 2004. This nine year position spanned his entire six years at Unitron and also, three years at the University of Western Ontario. Since 2005, he has also been instrumental in starting a new HIS program at Conestoga College, in Kitchener. Ted continues to give outside presentations on hearing loss and hearing aids.

The Cochlea, Hair Cells, and Compression

INTRODUCTION

This chapter covers some important concepts about the cochlea and its function, because these have everything to do with compression. In fact, this material is fundamental to a comprehensive understanding of compression in hearing aids.

The cochlea is described in general, broad strokes, with particular attention to the roles of the inner versus the outer hair cells. Each of these sets of hair cells does completely different things. We now know that the outer hair cells help the inner hair cells sense soft sounds and that the outer hair cells are usually damaged during normal wear and tear before the inner hair cells deteriorate. These different roles have ramifications for the types of compression that can be used in fitting people with hearing aids. The typical end result of outer hair cell damage is a sensorineural hearing loss of around 40 dB to 60 dB; this degree of hearing loss is consistent with the most common hearing loss today, which is presbycusis. The fitting of hearing aids for presbycusis may need to imitate the role of the outer hair cells in particular. This chapter outlines the problems posed by hair cell damage; Chapter 2 describes the nature of cochlear dead regions and implications for fitting hearing aids. Subsequent chapters discuss the goals of amplification for various degrees of hearing loss, hearing aid fitting methods, and the means of applying compression to different clinical populations.

A SKETCH OF COCHLEAR ANATOMY AND PHYSIOLOGY

Hearing aids, no matter how advanced their technology, whether they are analog or digital, cannot come close to restoring normal cochlear function. Put another way, pieces of plastic with amplifiers that are put into the ear, do not approach the glory of the normally functioning cochlea and its hair cells. The cochlea (from the Greek *kochlias* for snail shell) is one of the most complicated organs in the body, but its purpose can be explained in one sentence. It changes sound into electricity and electricity is the language the brain understands. The

An Unrolled Cochlea

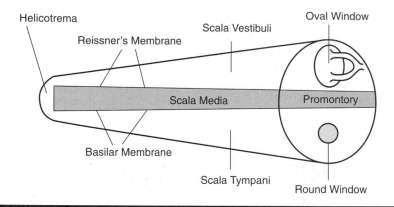

FIGURE 1–1   An unrolled cochlea shows the scala vestibuli and scala tympani wrapped around the scala media. These two chambers are continuous and are joined by the helicotrema. Therefore, they both share the same fluid, which is very different in composition than that inside the scala media. Note that the scala media is widest and thus has most mass at the smaller, pointed apex of the cochlea.

relative size of the cochlea in diagrams is often drawn far too large in relation to the size of the tympanic membrane. From lots of these erroneous diagrams, one would conceive of the cochlea as being about the size of an eyeball. This is fundamentally false; the cochlea is really quite small, about the size of the tip of your little finger. Its diameter is about that of the tympanic membrane. It has only 2½ turns in humans; in other mammals, the cochlea may look different. In the chinchilla, for example, the cochlea has 3½ turns.

As a complex organ, the cochlea and its functions are very difficult to comprehend. It might be easier to understand the relationships among its labyrinths, or chambers, and how they function if the snail-shaped cochlea could be unrolled into a straight line (Figure 1–1). Essentially, the cochlea consists of a soft-walled tube (membranous labyrinth) situated lengthwise inside a hard-walled cavity (bony labyrinth). The bony labyrinth is literally a hole inside the dense temporal bone of the skull, known as the petrous portion of the temporal bone. The word *petrous* originates from the Greek language, and has the same meaning as the name *Peter,* which means "hard, like a rock." The membranous labyrinth is closed at one end. It is actually narrowest at the wide base of the cochlea, and widest at the narrow apex. The membranous and bony labyrinths are each filled with fluids that have very different chemical compositions (Figure 1–1). The bony labyrinth (scala tympani and scala vestibuli) is filled with cerebral-spinal fluid, or "perilymph," which consists mostly of potassium, with less sodium. The membranous labyrinth (scala media) is filled with endolymph, consisting of the opposite ratio of mixture—mostly sodium with less potassium.

Note that the membranous labyrinth almost completely separates the bony labyrinth into an upper and a lower chamber. It is as if the bony labyrinth is bent

Cross Section of the Cochlea

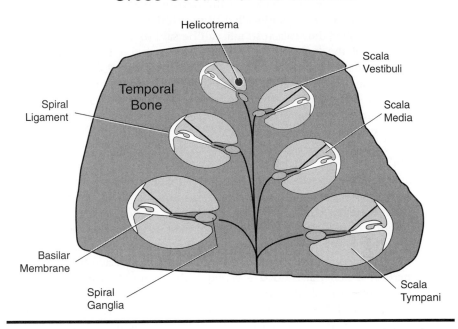

FIGURE 1–2 The human cochlea is often shown as if it exists as a snail-shaped presence, ready for easy excision and examination. Unlike the cochlea of many small mammals, however, the human cochlea is a labyrinth of coils completely embedded in bone (gray area in the figure). Therefore, the human cochlea is especially inaccessible. Note also, that the scala media is widest (and thus has most mass) at the smaller, pointed apex of the cochlea.

in the middle and folded in half. The membranous labyrinth is located between the upper and lower folds of the larger bony labyrinth, thus separating it into upper and lower portions. This relationship results in three chambers: a lower hard-walled chamber with a soft ceiling (scala tympani), a middle soft-walled chamber (scala media), and a higher hard-walled chamber with a soft floor (scala vestibuli). The upper and lower portions of the bony labyrinth are connected only at the bend, which is located at the apex or small tip of the cochlea (the helicotrema). The fluid in the scala vestibuli is thus continuous with the fluid inside the scala tympani.

In reality, the cochlea is coiled or rolled up, and therefore occupies a very small length in the skull, again, about the size of the tip of one's little finger. It might be a good idea to think of it as a coiled hole or labyrinth, augured into the petrous portion of the temporal bone of the skull, one of the densest bones in the body. One might as well look at a hole in the ground and then ask for the hole itself to be dug out, so it can be seen standing like a cup. It is no wonder that the human cochlea is very difficult to extract and show as a single unit.

A cross section of one coil of the rolled up cochlea reveals the three chambers described (Figure 1-2). The smallest chamber with the soft walls looks like a small triangle situated in the middle. Again, note how it is narrowest at the wide base of the cochlea and widest at the narrow apex. The top and bottom chambers correspond to the hard-walled labyrinth that is bent in half.

The top chamber, the scala vestibuli, can be said to "begin" at the oval window and "end" at the helicotrema. Similarly, the scala tympani begins at the round window of the cochlea and ends at the helicotrema. The hair cells of the cochlea are located in the middle chamber, the scala media. The "floor" upon which the hair cells stand in the cochlea is called the basilar membrane. It divides the bottom chamber, the scala tympani, from the middle chamber, or scala media. The basilar membrane runs along the whole length of the cochlea, from the base to the apex (Figure 1-1). When "unrolled," the basilar membrane is about 34 mm (about an inch) long (Yost, 2000).

Incoming sound, conducted by the middle ear bones that terminate at the oval window of the cochlea, moves the body of fluid that fills the scala vestibuli and scala tympani. The oval window (Figure 1-1) at the footplate of the middle ear stapes bone or ossicle, is the "entrance" to the cochlea; it consists of a small membrane that is pushed inward by incoming sound. The round window (Figure 1-1) is another small membrane on the cochlear surface that is situated below the oval window; it is not associated with any middle ear ossicle. When the oval window is pushed inward, the round window bulges outward. The resulting back and forth motion of fluid inside the scala vestibuli and scala tympani can be considered a "horizontal" movement. Incoming sounds of any frequency create this fluid motion. In fact, the horizontal back and forth fluid motion within the scala vestibuli and scala tympani occurs at the frequency of the sounds that created it (Yost, 2000); a 1000 Hz tone causes the footplate of the stapes to move back and forth 1000 times per second!

It is a "vertical" up and down motion of the basilar membrane, however, that bends the scala media at one particular place or another, and thus, stimulates the hair cells inside the scala media. Just exactly how or why the horizontal fluid motion translates into the vertical basilar membrane motion is quite a complex matter. Simply put, however, the basilar membrane, or floor of the scala media, has very different mass and stiffness properties at the base compared to the apex of the cochlea (Figure 1-1). According to Yost (2000), it is wider—and thus has more mass—at the narrow apex of the bony labyrinth, and narrower—and thus has less mass—at the wide base of the bony labyrinth! Also, the basilar membrane is quite flaccid at its wide end and stiffer at its narrow end. It is well known that low frequencies resonate with mass and less stiffness, while high frequencies resonate with less mass and more stiffness. These different physical properties cause the basilar membrane to resonate best at specific points along its length, depending on the many different frequencies of incoming sounds. Low, mid, and high frequencies of incoming sound each cause a maximal "vertical" indentation, at some unique spot along the length of the basilar membrane. This "vertical" motion is in the form of a *traveling wave,* with a peak occurring at one location or another along the length of the cochlea.

Recall that the outer walls of the scala vestibuli and scala tympani are hard bone (bony labyrinth), whereas the walls of the scala media are soft membranous (membranous labyrinth). Since this is the case, the only thing that can give or be displaced by the traveling wave peak is the soft scala media. The scala media is thus *indirectly* stimulated by incoming sound from the fluid movement within the scala vestibuli and scala tympani. Hair cells within the scala media are activated when incoming sound stimulates or bends the middle chamber at some particular place or point. When the traveling wave peak bends the scala media at the wide base of the cochlea and stimulates hair cells there, we hear high-frequency sounds; when the same happens at the apex, or narrow peak, of the cochlea, we hear low-frequency sounds. We will return to the traveling wave, and look at its unique asymmetrical shape, and the consequent upwards spread of masking later in this chapter.

As mentioned earlier, the tiny human cochlea is completely embedded in one of the hardest and most dense bones of the body, the petrous portion of the temporal bone (Figure 1–2). The cochlea is, therefore, quite inaccessible for physical examination, at least while a person is alive. The cochlea of the chinchilla has commonly been studied because, in this rodent, it sticks out into the middle ear space like a small honeycomb; this cochlea is much easier to excise and examine than that of a human. Only the relatively recent discovery of oto-acoustic emissions (OAEs) (Kemp, 1978) has provided us with a glimpse or a window into the real-time physiology, or function, of the human cochlea.

Oto-acoustic emissions have shown us that the function of the outer hair cells (OHCs) is very distinct from that of the inner hair cells (IHCs). The OHCs are mechanically motile; they actually stretch and shrink (Brownell, 1996). They are constantly in action, *amplifying soft incoming sounds* and *sharpening the peak of the traveling wave*. Because of this work, they emit a by-product: oto-acoustic emissions, which are like the hearing process "in reverse." Oto-acoustic emissions begin at the OHCs as *backwards-going* traveling waves, which strike the oval window and go *out from* the cochlea, *back* through the middle ear ossicular chain *to* the tympanic membrane. The eardrum in this case acts as a loudspeaker, converting the mechanical movement of the middle ear ossicles back into sound waves. It is bizarre but true that the ear can make sound as well as receive it!

Speaking of the middle ear, here may be a good place to posit the main reason why we have one in the first place. Most sounds to our ears arrive through the air and strike the eardrum. This airborne sound, however, has to penetrate the fluid-filled cochlea. As we all know, with our heads under water, our ears won't pick up much sound from someone talking at the side of the pool, outside of the water. Something has to increase the intensity or pressure level of the sound so it will be able to penetrate the water. That something is the middle ear. Sounds hitting the relatively large surface of the eardrum are all directed by the middle ear bones onto a much smaller surface area: the footplate of the stapes bone, and the smallest bone in the body. When force spread over a large area is directed onto a smaller area, the sound pressure (in decibels) becomes greater. This is the main role of the middle ear.

Back now to oto-acoustic emissions: Going backwards through the middle ear causes a reduction of sound pressure as the force of sound across the small footplate area of the stapes becomes dispersed over the larger area of the eardrum (Hall, 2000). This is why we cannot hear our own oto-acoustic emissions (or those of others!). Knowledge about the different IHC and OHC functions directly relates to compression in hearing aids. As is shown in later chapters, some types of compression are designed specifically to imitate the function of the OHCs. In this way, one can strive to amplify the wide variations of sound intensities to sound as natural as possible for persons with hearing loss.

INNER AND OUTER HAIR CELLS: STRUCTURE AND FUNCTION

Let's examine the IHCs and OHCs more closely. The IHCs are rounded or flask-like in shape like small pears. On each IHC, the 50 "hairs," or stereocilia, do not touch the tectorial membrane (see Figure 1–3). The IHCs communicate mostly with VIII cranial nerve fibers and terminate at the lower brainstem. More specifically, some 30,000 VIII cranial nerve fibers, mostly from some 3,000 IHCs in each cochlea exit the right and left cochleas and terminate at the right and left cochlear nuclei; these are located on the lower brainstem, where the medulla meets the pons.

Simple intuition suggests that, if things look different, they probably do different things. As Figure 1–3 shows, the IHCs and OHCs look different from each other and they do, indeed, have very different roles. The IHCs are mostly "afferent," which means that they send sound information *to* the brain (Brownell, 1996). Without IHCs, information about sound cannot be sent on to the brain and there is essentially no hearing. With damage to the IHCs, "brain-going" information is affected and a person may have difficulty understanding speech in quiet and especially with background noise (Killion, 1997b).

The OHCs are completely different. Unlike the IHCs, the 12,000 OHCs in each cochlea are cylindrical, or shaped like test tubes. On each OHC, some 100 "hairs," or stereocilia, are embedded in the bottom of the tectorial membrane (Figure 1–3). They receive communication from the low brainstem mostly through a bundle of neuron fibers, which leave the lower brainstem and terminate at the OHCs. These fibers are called the "olivo-cochlear bundle." The fibers of the olivo-cochlear bundle begin at the right and left superior olivary complexes in the low brainstem, run alongside of the afferent VIII nerve fibers, and end at the OHCs in both the opposite (crossed or contralateral) and same-side (uncrossed or ipsilateral) cochleas (Brownell, 1996).

The OHCs are "efferent," which means they take information *from* the brain back to the cochlea. They receive messages from the superior olivary nuclei in the lower brainstem (and probably higher centers as well). One should ask, then, how the superior olivary complexes get any afferent or incoming messages themselves, in order to communicate efferently with the OHCs. In addition, the OHCs have to react with incredible speed in order to mechanically

A Simple View of the Organ of Corti

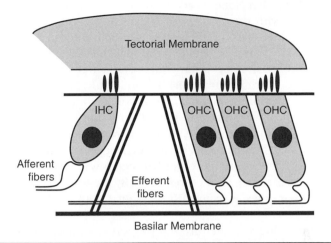

FIGURE 1–3   The inner (IHCs) and outer hair cells (OHCs) of the cochlea are very different in shape, and they also serve very different functions. The hairs or stereocilia of the OHCs are jammed into the underside of the tectorial membrane, whereas the stereocilia of the IHCs are not. The figure shows afferent fibers only at the IHCs and efferent fibers only at the OHCs, because, for the most part, these are the roles of the respective hair cells. In reality, however, a closer inspection would reveal that the arrangement is not so simple (some efferent fibers also are attached to the afferent fibers that terminate on the IHCs, and some afferent fibers are also attached to the OHCs themselves). When soft sounds enter the cochlea, the outer hair cells shrink, thus pulling down the tectorial membrane, so the stereocilia of the inner hair cells can be bent or sheared.

amplify and sharpen the traveling wave with incoming sounds. They must, therefore, have a *faster* way to receive any "call to action." We do know that the OHCs also receive chemical messages from inside the cochlea, which tell them to either elongate or shrink (Brownell, 1996; Yost, 2000). At this time no one really knows exactly how the whole afferent IHC and efferent OHC feedback loop, or system, works (Bobbin, 1996; Norris, 1996; Killion, 1996a).

The net effect of their mechanical action is to change the mechanical properties of the basilar membrane at specific spots. For soft incoming sounds, the OHCs play an especially strong role as they mechanically enable the IHCs to sense soft sounds and "sharpen" the peak of the traveling wave (Brownell, 1996). Without the OHCs, we would have a moderate degree (40–60 dB HL) of sensorineural hearing loss (Berlin, 1994). It follows that if someone has a severe hearing loss (e.g., 80 dB HL), then there is probably both IHC and OHC damage. More on this is discussed later. To truly appreciate the effect of the OHCs, we should first examine the passive traveling wave, without the action of the OHCs.

THE PASSIVE, ASYMMETRICAL TRAVELING WAVE

The name of a Hungarian Nobel Peace Prize winner, Georg von Bekesy, has become synonymous with the concept of a traveling wave peak that stimulates hair cells in specific areas along the basilar membrane. Recall that this cochlear membrane forms the boundary between the scala media and the scala tympani of the cochlea and is the "floor" upon which the hair cells are located. As mentioned earlier, the basilar membrane (34 mm in length) is relatively flaccid with more mass at the apex of the cochlea, and is stiff with less mass at the base of the cochlea. Specifically, it ranges from 0.42–0.65 mm in width at the narrow apex of the cochlea, and from 0.8–0.16 mm in width at the wider base of the cochlea (Figure 1–4). The small apex of the cochlea thus has more room, or "real estate," to accommodate about five outer hair cell rows than at the large base of the cochlea, where there are about three rows. By the way, this also is why there are *more* than three times as many OHCs (about 12,000) as IHCs (about 3000) in each cochlea.

Recall that it is due to these physical properties of mass and stiffness, that specific frequencies of sound produce traveling waves with peaks at specific places along the basilar membrane. High-frequency incoming sounds produce a traveling wave with a peak that stimulates the base and low-frequency incoming sounds produce a traveling wave with a peak that stimulates the apex of the cochlea. Again, the peak of this traveling wave movement is where the stereocilia of the inner hair cells bends or become sheared.

Figure 1–4 shows an exaggerated example of a traveling wave caused by low-frequency stimulation; its peak is located near the narrow cochlear apex, where the basilar membrane is widest. In truth, the size of the traveling wave is tiny. [To visualize a traveling wave in cadavers, von Bekesy (1960) had to present sounds at about 120 dB SPL] Note that the cochlear traveling wave is asymmetrical, with a "steep" wave front facing the low-frequency apex, and a relatively long, shallow "tail" sloping back towards the high-frequency base of the cochlea. The reason for the asymmetrical shape—and why the traveling wave has a peak in the first place—is because it *grows* and *slows* as it *goes* up the cochlea, until it reaches peak amplitude and stops. The traveling wave meets impedance along its travels up along the spiral of the cochlea. As it is forced to slow down along its "spiral" trip, its energy has to go somewhere; hence, its peak of "vertical" amplitude.

The asymmetry of the traveling wave has important implications for both audiometry and hearing aid fittings. If low-frequency hair cells are stimulated with a relatively large-amplitude traveling wave, then the entire basilar membrane moves and many hair cells from higher-frequency regions are also stimulated. On the other hand, if high-frequency hair cells are stimulated with a large-amplitude traveling wave, the low-frequency hair cells are not so easily stimulated. The asymmetry of the traveling wave is a cochlear explanation for what is commonly known as the "upward spread of masking." Classic masking experiments with psycho-physical tuning curves have also shown the relatively

Traveling Wave Along Basilar Membrane

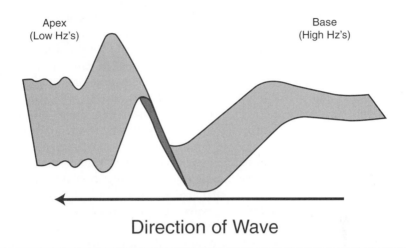

Apex
(Low Hz's)

Base
(High Hz's)

Direction of Wave

FIGURE 1–4   The basilar membrane is more narrow and stiff at the wide base of the cochlea; it is wider and less stiff at the narrow apex of the cochlea. These physical properties of mass and stiffness determine which hair cells are stimulated by incoming low-frequency or high-frequency sounds. The wider shape at the apex of the cochlea allows for more than the typical three rows of outer hair cells, often shown on diagrams.

greater efficiency of low-frequency versus high-frequency maskers (Bess & Humes, 2003). In short, low frequencies mask high frequencies better than high frequencies mask low frequencies. The rumble of a passing truck easily masks the peeping of a canary; however, the peeping of a canary is hard-pressed to mask the truck (no matter how loud that peeping is). The upward spread of masking can wreak havoc for the person with hearing aids when listening in background noise. More will be discussed on this topic later on in this chapter. The phenomenon of the upwards spread of masking is why hearing aid fitting methods often tend to prescribe relatively less amplification for the low frequencies than for the high frequencies (see Chapters 3 and 4).

Consider also, the audiometric testing of someone with a "reverse" hearing loss (moderate hearing loss for the low frequencies and normal hearing for the high frequencies); in this case, the actual, true low-frequency hearing loss could be worse than indicated on the audiogram (Thornton & Abbas, 1980; Halpin, Thornton, & Hasso, 1994). Due to the asymmetrical shape of the traveling wave, pure-tone testing of low frequencies, at levels greater than 50 dB HL may inadvertently stimulate the normally functioning high-frequency hair cells, causing the subject to respond. Similarly, when testing someone with a precipitous severe high-frequency SNHL, it is very possible that the high-frequency thresholds do not arise from surviving hair cells at the base of the cochlea. In fact, these thresholds might be "spurious artifacts," coming from the healthy hair cells representing the low frequencies at the apex of the cochlea. More will be discussed on the topic of cochlear dead regions in Chapter 2.

In summary, Von Bekesy (1960) described a passive traveling wave with a rounded peak, but recall that he used mostly cadavers in his studies, which of course have dead hair cells. More recent studies have shown that the same dull, rounded peak is also found in cochleas that have damaged hair cells (Brownell, 1996). A passive traveling wave with a dull, rounded peak presents problems when trying to figure out how the cochlea "fine-tunes" for frequencies that are close together. For example, if humans can hear frequencies from 20 to 20,000 Hz, then how can a dull, rounded traveling wave allow us to distinguish the difference between, say, 500 Hz and 520 Hz? Some thought might lead one to question the gross nature of hair cell stimulation with such a rounded peak. How does the cochlea do precise fine-tuning? According to Brownell (1996), a colleague of von Bekesy's (Gold, 1948), had proposed that the OHCs had an active role in sharpening the traveling wave peak, but this explanation was dismissed by von Bekesy from lack of evidence. The VIII nerve was known to have sharp tuning curves, and von Bekesy believed that a fine frequency resolution thus took place further "up" the auditory system chain of command. A fascinating historical account of these developments in cochlear discoveries can be found in a textbook on oto-acoustic emissions by Hall (2000).

Imagine the real-life implications of OHC damage resulting in a dull, rounded traveling wave; with poorer frequency resolution, or a reduced ability to distinguish between frequencies that are close together, is it not reasonable to suppose one will experience increased difficulty in listening to speech in a noisy environment? No wonder people who wear hearing aids complain so bitterly about background noise! Hearing aids are merely amplifiers; they cannot actively sharpen a traveling wave peak like the OHCs do.

OHCs AND ACTIVE TRAVELING WAVE

The concept of the active versus the passive cochlea is relatively new; only since around 1990 has this view of the cochlea become a real part of the clinician's knowledge base. Through the discovery of oto-acoustic emissions, we now know that the OHCs do indeed have an *active* role in cochlear mechanics.

An active (as opposed to passive) traveling wave with OHC involvement is shown in Figure 1-5. In this example, the low-frequency hair cells are receiving most of the traveling wave excitation. The peak of the traveling wave is the site of greatest hair cell stimulation, but without the OHCs, the peak is rounded. Given a hearing range of from about 20 to 20,000 Hz, such a dull, rounded traveling wave peak stimulates many different frequencies at once.

By themselves, without the action of the OHCs, the IHCs are stimulated by the motion of endolymph fluid in the scala media. This only occurs with incoming

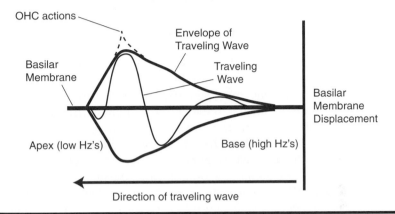

FIGURE 1–5   The basilar membrane is the "floor" upon which the inner and outer hair cells are situated. On the left are the low-frequency hair cells at the apex of the cochlea; on the right are the high-frequency hair cells at the base of the cochlea. The traveling wave bends the basilar membrane, which in turn excites the hair cells. Note that the envelope of the traveling wave is asymmetrical. Without the action of the outer hair cells, the traveling wave has a dull, rounded peak. This passive traveling wave peak stimulates many adjacent frequencies simultaneously. The increase in amplitude and sharpening of the peak is accomplished with the action of the outer hair cells. The amplitude increase enables one to hear soft sounds, and the sharpening increases the ability to distinguish between frequencies that are close together.

sounds of 40 dB to 60 dB SPL or more (Bobbin, 1996; Killion, 1996a; Moore, 2001). With softer incoming sounds, like 10 dB SPL, the OHCs are somehow stimulated to be mechanically motile (perhaps through chemical messages from within the cochlea, as mentioned earlier), thus helping the IHCs sense soft sounds. Without the OHCs, the IHCs can sense sounds from about 40 dB to 60 dB SPL up to the level of physical sensation or total loudness discomfort; by themselves, the IHCs cannot sense sounds below these levels. Damage to the OHCs thus implies a hearing loss of 40 dB to 60 dB, and this is often the degree of hearing loss found with presbycusis.

In addition to amplifying soft incoming sounds for the IHCs, the mechanical action of the OHCs also "sharpens" the peak of the traveling wave (Brownell, 1996). With their mechanical stretching and shrinking movements, these motile OHCs temporarily alter the physical properties of the basilar membrane around both sides of the passive peak of the traveling wave, mechanically forcing the peak into a sharper point. This, in turn, increases our ability to distinguish between frequencies that are close together. A passive traveling wave with a dull, rounded peak may not enable one to distinguish among frequencies that are close together. Again, is it any wonder then that the person with OHC damage may have poorer speech discrimination ability, especially within a noisy environment?

The whole active cochlear mechanism is extremely complex. As mentioned earlier, think of the speed at which the OHCs have to move to influence the reception of sounds by the IHCs; the OHCs must be able to move or react very quickly. In fact, the OHCs do have the ability to move faster than any muscle (Brownell, 1996). With soft incoming sounds, the OHCs shrink. Because their stereocilia are actually embedded in the tectorial membrane, the OHCs pull the membrane down when they shrink, and this shortens the gap between the tectorial membrane and the tips of the IHC stereocilia. When the tips of the IHC stereocilia can touch the tectorial membrane, they can be bent or sheared and thereby send sound information to the brain. So for soft sound inputs, the OHCs mechanically help the IHC stereocilia to make contact so they can be sheared or bent by the tectorial membrane. In Figure 1-5, it appears that the OHCs literally "heighten" and "sharpen" the peak of the traveling wave. Note also, that the *active* traveling wave in Figure 1-5 has an asymmetrical shape that is reminiscent of the tuning curves of VIII nerve fibers.

Each of the 30,000 VIII nerve fibers has its own specific tuning curve. The tuning curve for any one VIII nerve fiber shows that the fiber in question is frequency specific. At some specific frequency, the least intensity is required to make that specific neuron fiber fire. This is the "characteristic" frequency of the specific neuron fiber. At progressively lower or higher frequencies, greater and greater intensities are required to get that same neuron to fire. The same required intensity, however, increases far more rapidly for frequencies above the characteristic frequency than for frequencies below it. In this way, the tuning curve for any specific VIII nerve fiber is asymmetrical.

Psycho-physical tuning curves, mentioned earlier in this chapter, have a similar asymmetrical shape (Bess & Humes, 2003). These tuning curves show how much masking intensity is required at different frequencies in order to behaviorally mask some specific signal tone frequency. It is important not to confuse this kind of masking with the typical contralateral masking done in clinical audiometric testing; that type of masking is done to eliminate the non-test ear from the routine audiometric test. The type of masking done to derive psycho-physical tuning curves is delivered ipsilaterally, or else in a sound field to both ears, and it is performed mainly by researchers interested in psychoacoustics. Narrow bands of masking are usually used because this helps the subject distinguish between the signal tone and the masker itself.

Psycho-physical tuning curves illustrate that the best masker is one close to the signal tone frequency. As with the VIII nerve tuning curves, at progressively lower or higher frequencies, more and more intensity is required for the masking noise to effectively mask the signal tone frequency in question. However, the required intensity for the noise to mask the signal tone frequency increases far more rapidly for higher frequencies than for lower frequencies. The asymmetrical traveling wave shown in Figures 1-4, 1-5, VIII nerve tuning curves, and psycho-physical tuning curves all point to the phenomenon known as "the upward spread of masking;" the fact that low frequencies mask high frequencies better than vice versa. With outer hair cell damage, the traveling wave loses its sharp peak and becomes more dull and rounded, the VIII nerve fiber tuning curves become wider and lose the sharpness of their characteristic frequencies, and consequently, the psycho-physical tuning curves showing the effects of masking are also widened. These would all imply that the person has a harder time distinguishing between frequencies that are close together. They also show that, when listening to a signal sound, he/she is more easily masked by surrounding frequencies. The interested reader is encouraged to consult Yost (2000).

In summary, the OHCs have a twofold purpose: (1) they amplify soft incoming sounds below 40 dB to 60 dB SPL, allowing the IHCs to sense them, and (2) they also fine-tune the frequency resolution of the cochlea (Figure 1-5). With damage to the OHCs, we have a corresponding loss of these functions. As mentioned earlier, this results in a 40 dB to 60 dB (mild-to-moderate) sensorineural hearing loss (SNHL). If the hearing loss is greater than mild-to-moderate in degree, then there is probably both IHC and OHC damage. Of course, it should not be presumed that for all those with SNHL, damage occurs strictly to the OHCs before any damage occurs to the IHCs. There is some intersection between the damage that occurs to both sets of hair cells, and furthermore, this intersection differs among those with the same degree of SNHL In general, however, damage to OHCs tends to occur before damage to IHCs.

Imagine now what goes on within the cochleas of someone with a moderate degree (or more) of SNHL when he/she is wearing hearing aids: With amplification, a small traveling wave with a dull, rounded peak is increased to become a larger traveling wave with a dull, rounded peak (Figure 1-6). In short, hearing amplification alone does not result in normal hearing. Amplification can only achieve the first role of the OHCs, namely, increasing the size of the traveling wave peak, especially for soft incoming sounds. Hearing aids cannot sharpen the peak of the traveling wave. If they could, practicing clinicians would not constantly hear the complaints of difficulty listening to speech in noise. For improved speech reception performance in noise, the signal-to-noise ratio (SNR) has to be increased; that is, the decibel level of speech would have to be increased relative to the decibel level of background noise. With an increased SNR, those with damaged hair cells can still find improvement for their speech reception performance in background noise. Directional microphones in hearing aids, and to a lesser degree, digital noise reduction (see Chapter 8), can serve to more specifically address these kinds of complaints.

The Traveling Wave: Naturally Sharpened vs Aided

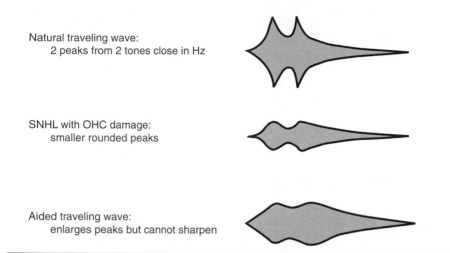

Natural traveling wave:
    2 peaks from 2 tones close in Hz

SNHL with OHC damage:
    smaller rounded peaks

Aided traveling wave:
    enlarges peaks but cannot sharpen

FIGURE 1–6   These idealized, schematic shapes represent three traveling wave envelopes. The top shows a theoretical schematic of a normal traveling wave envelope, resulting from stimulation of two tones close together but different in frequency. The middle shows a traveling wave envelope resulting from the same stimulation; however, due to outer hair cell damage, this one is reduced in amplitude and its peaks are rounded. The bottom shows what would happen with amplification. The original wave size has been restored, but the peaks are still rounded. In other words, the ability to distinguish between frequencies close together has not been restored. This would also imply that the ability to separate speech from background noise has not been improved with amplification alone.

DAMAGED HAIR CELLS AND HEARING LOSS

To contrast normal and damaged hair cells, look at the electron microscope photographs in Figures 1-7 and 1-8. Healthy normal IHCs and OHCs are seen in Figure 1-7. The 40 to 60 stereocilia on each of the 3000 IHCs in each cochlea are arranged in shallow "Vs." The 100 or so stereocilia on each of the 12,000 OHCs in each cochlea are arranged like "horseshoes" in three or more rows.

Figure 1-8 shows damaged hair cells. Note that the damage is mostly confined to the OHCs. Loss of outer hair cells causes loss of OHC function, which results in more passive, dull and less active, sharp traveling waves. In audiometry, this translates into mild-to-moderate SNHL. Because the OHCs are very mechanical (i.e., they move a lot), they use lots of oxygen. These highly mobile hair cells are very sensitive to the insults that life throws at them over the years of one's existence. Most hair cell damage thus begins with the OHCs and later on is evident in the IHCs (Willott, 1991). If the SNHL is about 50 dB HL or less in degree, it can usually be assumed that the damage is mostly confined to the

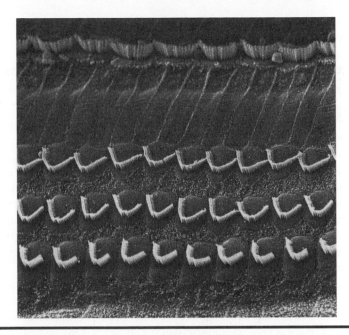

FIGURE 1–7   An electron microscope photograph of normal, healthy human inner and outer hair cells. Note. From *The Biology of Hearing and Deafness* (p. 21), by R. Harrison, 1988, Springfield IL: Charles C Thomas, Publisher. Copyright 1988 by Charles C Thomas, Publisher. Reprinted with permission.

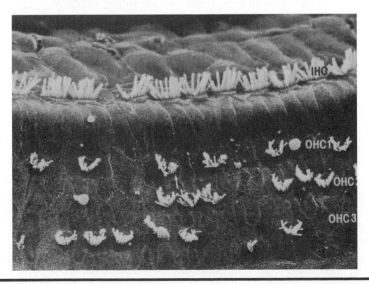

FIGURE 1–8   An electron microscope photograph of damaged hair cells. Most of the damage is confined to the outer hair cells. Note. From *The Ear: Some Notes on Structure and Function* (p. 12), by H. Engstrom and B. Engstrom, 1988, Vaerloese, Denmark: Widex. Copyright by Widex. Reprinted with permission.

outer hair cells. If the hearing loss is, for example, 80 dB HL, then it is safe to assume that the damage involves both IHCs and OHCs.

Presbycusis: The Most Common Type of Hearing Loss

The word *presbycusis* is composed of two Greek words: *presby,* which means "elders," and *cusis,* which means "hearing." Presbycusis is reminiscent of the word *presbyterian,* which means "church of the elders," and *presbyopia,* which means "vision of the elders."

Presbycusis, or hearing loss found in aging ears, manifests itself as mild-to-moderate SNHL, and it is by far the most common type of hearing loss in our society today. About 80% of the people living in the United States with hearing loss have presbycusis (Hull, 1995). Demographics show that as the baby boom generation ages, there is a large "bubble," or segment, of people who are increasing in age and so the average age of our population is also increasing. Therefore, we should expect to see an increase of clients having presbycusis in the future.

Most presbycusis results in mild-to-moderate SNHL, which is consistent with OHC damage. People with presbycusis often have a hearing loss that is mild in degree for the low frequencies and moderate in degree for the high frequencies. Jerger, Chmiel, Stach, and Spretnjak (1993) compared hearing loss configurations in men and women between the ages of 50 and 89 years. They found that, in general, men often have a more steeply sloping hearing loss than women, with a greater degree of hearing loss in the high frequencies and less hearing loss in the low frequencies. For women, the greater hearing loss in the low frequencies might result from degeneration of the stria vascularis, which affects blood supply to the cochlear hair cells. For men, the greater hearing loss in the high frequencies might show the interaction of noise-induced hearing loss (NIHL) and presbycusis.

NIHL also causes damage to the OHCs (Engstrom & Engstrom, 1988), especially when the noise to which the person is exposed is constant. However, according to Borg, Canlon, and Engstrom (1995) and Killion (1997b), sudden, sharp noises like loud gunshots will cause both IHC and OHC damage. As mentioned earlier, OHC damage may result in some trouble understanding speech in background noise; but the IHCs send most sound information to the brain. If these IHCs are damaged, then the message to the brain is "garbled," resulting in dramatically increased difficulty separating speech from background noise, even when clients are properly aided (see also Chapter 3)! Noise in our society is gradually becoming more of an issue for concern, especially as general awareness of NIHL filters through to the general public.

Hearing Aids for the Damaged Cochlea

Figure 1–9 is a verbal analogy of the results of normal versus damaged hair cells as seen in Figures 1–7 and 1–8, respectively. Hearing aids must meet a daunting goal in trying to imitate the action of the normal cochlea. Unfortunately, this cannot be done. At present trying to restore normal hearing with hearing aids is

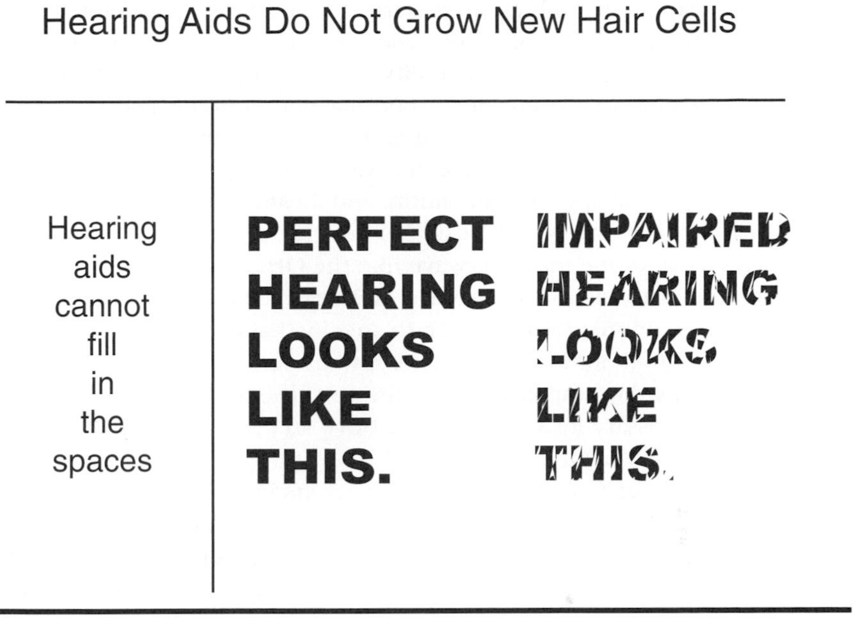

Hearing Aids Do Not Grow New Hair Cells

Hearing aids cannot fill in the spaces	PERFECT HEARING LOOKS LIKE THIS.	IMPAIRED HEARING LOOKS LIKE THIS.

FIGURE 1–9   A verbal illustration of the normal and damaged hair cells shown in Figures 1-7 and 1-8. With normal hearing, there are many hair cells. With hearing loss, hair cells are damaged and/or there are fewer cells. Can amplification of fewer hair cells possibly imitate the action of many hair cells? At most, hearing aids will make the white areas of the figure (right side) become whiter and the black areas become darker, but they cannot fill in the spaces. Note. Adapted from a poster. Copyright held by The Canadian Hearing Society, Toronto, Ontario, Canada. Adapted with permission.

like trying to pick up needles with mittens on. The amplified sound must get through the middle ear to the cochlea and stimulate damaged or missing hair cells. We are not simply sending amplified sound to intact hair cells; nor are we fitting mostly conductive hearing loss. If we were, hearing aid fittings would be more straightforward, perhaps a bit more like fitting eyeglasses.

Hearing aids cannot grow new hair cells. Although a few experiments have shown that we can reproduce hair cells in birds (Ryals, 1995), as we go higher up in the animal kingdom, hair cells are more difficult to reproduce. When we can grow new hair cells, hearing aids will become extinct and the reader (and author) will be looking for other work. However, because that will not likely happen in the near future, emphasis needs to be placed on developing the best hearing aids possible.

Amplification alone increases audibility of sounds but does not come close to the majesty and wonder of the healthy cochlea. As we all know, hearing aids and people too often mix like oil and water. Amplification is only one part of the story for improving the quality of life for those with hearing loss; increased SNR is the other part. Only with an increased SNR can those with diminished frequency resolution ability enjoy increased speech reception performance in background noise. To this end, the ability to hear speech in the midst of background noise can be improved with directional microphones, and listening comfort in noise can be enhanced with digital noise reduction.

The results of a sharpened traveling wave can be intuitively surmised: It is probable that frequency discrimination and hearing in noise are improved (or normal) with a sharpened peak. No hearing aid presently available can sharpen the peak of the traveling wave like the OHCs do. But as we have seen, the OHCs are also known to increase cochlear sensitivity by at least 40 dB (Killion, 1996a). Moore (2001) goes on to specify that the "gain" provided by the OHCs is about 50 dB for low frequencies and up to 65 dB for the high frequencies. For the IHCs, the "amplification," or lifting of the traveling wave peak by the OHCs, is not necessary for sound inputs above 40 to some 65 dB SPL (i.e., they need no help from the OHCs).

Hair cell damage (mostly to the OHCs) results in the most common type of hearing loss—a moderate sensorineural hearing loss (SNHL), where soft sounds below conversational speech (50–65 dB HL) are inaudible, and yet 90 dB to 100 dB HL sounds are perceived as loud, just as they would to someone with normal hearing. For this person, hearing aids should amplify the soft sounds by a lot, and amplify louder sounds by progressively less and less. Hearing aids that accomplish this are specifically intended to imitate what the outer hair cells once did; these are hearing aids with wide dynamic range compression (WDRC). The OHCs begin their work for sounds below 50 dB to 65 dB SPL; hence, the kneepoint of WDRC is most often found at input levels of around 50 dB as well. Much more on this topic of compression will be discussed in Chapter 5. The cochlea is a nonlinear organ. The softer the input, the more it amplifies. Perhaps this is a rationale for using nonlinear amplification. Recent knowledge about the function of the cochlea has everything to do with compression in hearing aids.

SUMMARY

- The OHCs sharpen the peak of the traveling wave and amplify soft incoming sounds below approximately 40 dB to 50 dB SPL. With hearing aids today, we can imitate only the second of these functions.

- The OHCs are mechanical in nature, they use a lot of oxygen, and they are usually the first to die or be damaged. Loss of the OHCs results in a mild-to-moderate degree of hearing loss. If hearing loss is severe, there is probably damage to the IHCs as well as the OHCs.

- The most common type of hearing loss today is presbycusis, which is typically mild to moderate in degree. For this population, we need to try to imitate OHC function, and to do so we must amplify soft sounds by a lot and intense sounds by little or nothing at all.

REVIEW QUESTIONS

1. The cochlea and vestibular system are located in the:
   a. mastoid portion of the temporal bone
   b. petrous portion of the temporal bone
   c. mastoid portion of the petrous bone
   d. temporal portion of the mastoid bone

2. The scala tympani is associated with the _____; the scala vestibuli is associated with the:
   a. oval window / round window
   b. stria vascularis / spiral ligament
   c. round window / oval window
   d. spiral ligament / stria vascularis

3. How many rows of inner hair cells typically exist at the apex of the cochlea?
   a. one   c. five
   b. three   d. 10

4. The front of the passive cochlear traveling wave is _____ and faces the _____
   a. steep / base
   b. long / base
   c. long / apex
   d. steep / apex

5. The traveling wave has a:
   a. long, shallow tail and a short steep front
   b. short, steep tail and a long, shallow front
   c. symmetrical shape for both the tail and front
   d. shape that looks just like the sound that created it

6. Intense low Hz sounds create a traveling wave that stimulates:
   a. only the hair cells at the base of the cochlea
   b. hair cells mostly at the base of the cochlea but also some at the apex
   c. only the hair cells at the apex of the cochlea
   d. hair cells mostly at the apex of the cochlea but also some at the base

7. Von Bekesy, who discovered the traveling wave, thought it had a:
   a. symmetrical shape
   b. sharpened peak
   c. dull, rounded peak
   d. short, steep tail and a long, shallow front

8. The discovery of OAEs is attributed to:
   a. von Bekesy
   b. Kemp
   c. Gold
   d. none of the above

9. Outer hair cells become active for incoming sounds below ___ dB SPL.
   a. 0-20
   b. 20-40
   c. 40-60
   d. 60-80

10. The following statement is true about the outer hair cells; they:
    a. are located in the scala tympani
    b. are fewer in number than the inner hair cells
    c. decrease our frequency resolution
    d. increase our frequency resolution

RECOMMENDED READINGS

Hall, III, J. W. (2000). *Handbook of oto-acoustic emissions.* San Diego: Singular Publishing Inc.

Yost, W. A. (2000). *Fundamentals of hearing: An introduction* (4th ed.). San Diego: Academic Press.

REFERENCES

Berlin, C. I. (1994). When outer hair cells fail, use correct circuitry to simulate their function. *The Hearing Journal, 47*(4): 43.

Bess, F. H., & Humes, L. E. (2003). *Audiology: The fundamentals* (3rd ed.). Baltimore: Williams and Wilkins.

Bobbin, R. P. (1996). Chemical receptors on outer hair cells and their molecular mechanisms. In C. I. Berlin (Ed.), *Hair cells and hearing aids* (pp. 29-56). San Diego: Singular Publishing Group, Inc.

Borg, E., Canlon, B., & Engstrom, B. (1995). Noise induced hearing loss: Literature review and experiments in rabbits. *Scandinavian Audiology, 24*(Suppl. 40): 117-125.

Brownell, W. E. (1996). Outer hair cell electromotility and otoacoustic emissions. In C. I. Berlin (Ed.), *Hair cells and hearing aids* (pp. 3-28). San Diego: Singular Publishing Group, Inc.

Engstron, H., & Engstrom, B. (1988, June). *The Ear*. Uppsala Sweden: Widex.

Gold, T. (1948). The physical basis of the action of the cochlea. *Proceedings of the Royal Society of London, Biological Science, 135,* 492–498.

Halpin, Thornton, & Hasso. (1994). Low-frequency sensorineural hearing loss: Clinical evaluation and implications for hearing aid fitting. *Ear and Hearing, 15*(1): 71–81.

Hall, III, J. W. (2000). *Handbook of oto-acoustic emissions*. San Diego CA: Singular Publishing Group, Inc.

Hull, R. H. (1995). Hearing in Aging. San Diego, Singular Publishing Group Inc.

Jerger, J., Chmiel, R., Stach, B., & Spretnjak, J. (1993). Gender affects audiometric shape in presbycusis. *Journal of the American Academy of Audiology,* 4: 42–49.

Kemp, D. T. (1978). Stimulated acoustic emissions from within the human auditory system. *Journal of the Acoustical Society of America, 64,* 1386–1391.

Killion, M. C., (1997a). "I can hear what people say, but I can't understand them." *The Hearing Review, 4*(12): 8–14.

Killion, M. C. (1997b). The SIN report: Circuits haven't solved the hearing-in-noise problem. *The Hearing Journal, 50*(10): 28–34.

Moore, B. C. J. (2001). Dead regions in the cochlea: Diagnosis, perceptual consequences, and amplification for the fitting of hearing aids. Trends in Amplification, 5(1): 1–34.

Norris, C. H. (1996). Cochlear outer hair cells vis-a-vis semicircular canal type II hair cells. In C. I. Berlin (Ed.), *Hair cells and hearing aids* (pp. 3–28). San Diego: Singular Publishing Group, Inc.

Ryals, B. M., (1995). Hair cell regeneration: Is it just for the birds? *The Hearing Journal, 48*(7): 10–83.

Thornton, A., & Abbas, P. (1980). Low-frequency hearing loss: Perception of filtered speech, psychophysical tuning curves, and masking. *Journal of the Acoustical Society of America, 67,* 623–643.

Von Bekesy, G. (1960). *Experiments in hearing*. New York: McGraw-Hill.

Yost, W. A. (2000). *Fundamentals of hearing: An introduction* (4th ed.). San Diego: Academic Press, Inc.

Willott, J. F. (1991). *Aging and the auditory system: Anatomy, physiology, and psychophysics*. San Diego: Singular Publishing Group, Inc.

2

The Cochlear Dead Spot Concept
Implications for Hearing Aid Fittings

INTRODUCTION

The cochlea is the "retina" of the ear; it changes sound into electricity, and electricity is the "language" the brain understands. However, just as dead areas of the retina can make holes in one's visual field, dead hair cell spots or regions within the cochlea can produce dead frequency regions of hearing sensitivity. At these frequencies, hearing aid amplification does little or no good at all. The purpose of this chapter is to describe how these dead areas can be identified, to illustrate what kinds of audiograms are often associated with cochlear dead spots, and indicate some implications of cochlear dead regions in subsequent hearing aid fittings.

Cochlear dead spots occur where there is complete destruction to the inner hair cells. As mentioned in Chapter 1, the inner hair cells are the transducers of the cochlea, while the outer hair cells serve to enable the inner hair cells to sense soft incoming sounds. According to Moore (2001), the outer hair cells provide amplification or "gain" of about 50 dB for the low frequencies and about 65 dB for the high frequencies. Beyond these decibel levels, additional inner hair cell damage can only result in another 25 dB to 30 dB of hearing loss. As a result, cochlear dead regions are to be associated with hearing loss of 90 dB beyond normal thresholds, in the mid to high frequencies, and greater than 75 dB to 80 dB beyond normal thresholds in the low frequencies.

A recently developed clinical procedure to identify cochlear dead regions (Moore, 2001; Moore, Glasburg, & Stone, 2004) is described in this chapter. The procedure, from Moore and colleagues (2004) at Cambridge University, is known as the Threshold Equalizing Noise (TEN) test. It has been put on a CD and is available for clinical implementation. The assessment of cochlear dead hair cell regions—and the implications for hearing aid fittings—remains a fairly hot topic at conferences for audiologists and for hearing instrument specialists. The most interesting thing about the whole cochlear dead spots concept is not the TEN test, nor is it the CD itself. In the author's opinion (Venema, 2003), the

Upward Spread of Masking

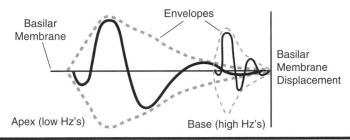

Intense *Low-Hz* traveling wave moves *entire* Basilar Membrane

Intense *High-Hz* traveling waves moves Basilar Membrane *only at base*

Basilar Membrane

Envelopes

Basilar Membrane Displacement

Apex (low Hz's)

Base (high Hz's)

FIGURE 2–1   The traveling wave is asymmetric in shape. Soft, high-frequency stimulation would result in a small traveling wave at the base of the cochlea (right), which would easily be overcome or masked by the wave resulting from intense low-frequency stimulation at the apex (left). The reverse would not be true; intense high-frequency stimulation would result in a traveling wave confined to the base of the cochlea (right), and thus, it would not interfere with the wave resulting from soft low-frequency stimulation (left).

most fascinating thing by far is the rationale behind the TEN test and the education it demands; in order to understand how the test works, one is forced to appreciate cochlear physiology.

In order to understand the TEN test for cochlear dead spots, it is essential to keep in mind the asymmetrical shape of the traveling wave envelope, with a long sloping "tail" towards the wide high-frequency base of the cochlea, and its relatively steep front facing the low-frequency apex of the cochlea (Figure 2-1). The (1) asymmetrical traveling wave shape is also reflected in the shapes of (2) VIII nerve fiber tuning curves and in (3) psycho-physical (behavioral) tuning curves. All of these three concepts were discussed earlier in Chapter 1.

WHAT ARE COCHLEAR DEAD REGIONS?

We learned in Chapter 1 that outer hair cells help the inner hair cells sense soft incoming sounds. Dead regions in the cochlea occur when inner hair cells are completely destroyed or absent in certain places along the basilar membrane. Recall that the snail-shaped human cochlea has 2 ½ turns or coils. Imagine the rolled-up cochlea to be "unrolled," as in Chapter 1, Figure 1-1. When unrolled, it is slightly over an inch long (about 34 mm). Inside this unrolled cochlea is a smaller tube (scala media); it is here that the hair cells grow, along the whole length, from end to end. Now imagine there to be an area about the width of your pinkie fingernail—it could be anywhere on the scala media—where there are no inner hair cells. That area would be a cochlear dead spot. In such a dead region, there is no hearing sensitivity at all. The person is totally deaf at those frequencies.

Symmetrical dead regions occur when the area of completely missing hair cells is located in exactly the same place (or contained in the same frequency boundaries) within both cochleas of the individual. Of course, the person's audiogram would show symmetrical sensorineural hearing loss (SNHL) too. If, on the other hand, the dead regions were located in different locations inside the cochlea, they would be asymmetrical and, accordingly, the person would show SNHL at different frequencies and would have an asymmetrical audiogram.

Cochlear dead regions can be hereditary or acquired (Venema & McSpaden, 2004). Hereditary cochlear dead regions can appear in a variety of audiometric shapes or configurations. Any of these can have a wide variety of severity and can be symmetrical or asymmetrical. Some audiogram configurations associated with cochlear dead regions are: low-frequency SNHL rising towards better hearing in the mid and high frequencies (the reverse audiogram), a mid-frequency hearing loss with better low- and high-frequency hearing (the "cookie-bite" audiogram), and the precipitous severe, high-frequency audiogram. Sometimes hereditary SNHL can result in a really jagged or bizarre-looking audiogram shape. The author recalls testing a young woman with hereditary SNHL that sloped rather steeply from moderate to profound in one ear; and in the other ear, she seemed to have an "island" of good hearing at 1000 Hz, with poorer hearing on either side frequencies!

An example of an acquired cochlear dead region is that of severe noise-induced hearing loss (NIHL). It is of interest to note *why* the NIHL occurs mostly around 4000 Hz; basically between 3000 to 6000 Hz. Noise-caused damage tends to affect hair cells that represent frequencies about a half an octave above the noise that caused it (Yost, 2000). To understand why NIHL occurs between 3000 and 6000 Hz, it may help to look at the resonance of the adult outer ear canal, which stretches from about 1500 Hz to around 4000 Hz, and has a 10 dB to 20 dB peak at around 2700 Hz. This broad peak of added resonance, when moved "up" a half an octave, can result in damage to cochlear hair cells representing frequencies between 3000 and 6000 Hz. The typical NIHL audiogram then improves beyond 6000 Hz because the resonance of the outer ear canal, which gives the 10 dB to 20 dB of extra dose of noise in the first place, drops off just beyond 4000 Hz (a half an octave lower). Over a prolonged length of exposure to noise, NIHL can become so severe that it results in completely dead high-frequency hair cells, which in turn cause a severe-to-profound precipitous high-frequency SNHL.

NIHL can be symmetrical or asymmetrical. Asymmetrical NIHL will more likely be seen in hunters, truck drivers, or anyone else who has been exposed to more excessive noise on one side than on the other. Right-handed rifle hunters often have more NIHL for the left ear, because when the hunter holds the rifle and takes aim, the head acts as a barrier or head shadow, blocking some of the sound from hitting the right ear; the left gets most of the "bang." It's vice versa for the left-handed hunter.

Here's an aside: Much of the noise from gunshot is not from the gunpowder exploding; rather, it's from the bullet breaking the sound barrier! Gun silencers seen on movies actually slow the bullet down, preventing it from breaking the sound barrier. That's why the movies almost always show silencers being used at close range!

THE TEN TEST CD: DESCRIPTION, PROCEDURE, AND RATIONALE

Moore (2001), a prominent Cambridge University researcher in areas of psychoacoustics, has developed a test to clinically identify cochlear dead spots; it is called the Threshold Equalizing Noise (TEN) test. The TEN test comes on a CD that can be played over a two-channel audiometer. The CD is available from Moore's lab and the website is given at the end of this chapter. The CD has separate tracks that play pure tones, in octave and sometimes mid-octave audiometric frequencies, as well as a *single broad band masking noise* that encompasses all of these frequencies. This masking noise is the TEN. It is quite different from the narrow bands of noise used in our audiometers. The pure tones and the TEN must be directed towards the same ear (ipsilaterally), and this can only be done with a two-channel audiometer. The intensity of the tones as well as the noise can then be separately adjusted by way of the intensity controls on the audiometer, and both of these are sent to either the right or left ear. The general procedure of the TEN test involves first testing for thresholds of the pure tones from the CD, and then retesting the same ear for thresholds while the masking noise is presented into the *same* ear (ipsilateral masking).

The CD is plugged into the tape inputs of the audiometer, and pure-tone thresholds are obtained from the client in quiet through the headphones. Insert headphones are generally recommended because they have a flatter frequency response than circumaural headphones. Behavioral thresholds are then retested with ipsilaterally presented TEN. Sufficient TEN must be presented in order to just mask the thresholds of interest—frequencies where cochlear dead hair cells are suspected. For example, with a sloping high-frequency hearing loss, where one might suspect high-frequency cochlear dead regions, the TEN intensity level should be enough to just mask the high-frequency thresholds. With the TEN being presented, retest all the hearing thresholds again, and then compare the masked thresholds to the unmasked thresholds. The broadband TEN would, of course, elevate all thresholds at which it is audible. That is, it should raise all thresholds at least up to the dB level of the TEN. Moore (2001) has suggested that with ipsilaterally presented TEN, those thresholds that are of interest or under suspicion of arising from cochlear dead hair cell regions could very well end up being a few (2–3) dB above the TEN intensity level. This finding might arise from the increased effects of masking upon frequency regions of the cochlea where there is damage confined mostly to the outer hair cells. This would not be considered a cochlear dead hair cell region.

Suspect dead inner hair cells, however, at frequencies where the ipsilateral TEN increases the thresholds to a dB level that is at least 10 dB greater than the TEN intensity level itself. This +10 dB shift (relative to the TEN dB level) is Moore's criteria for assessing the presence of cochlear dead hair cell regions. Such a large threshold increase means that for the pure-tone frequencies of interest, the unmasked and masked thresholds actually arise from remote healthy hair cells that do not represent the frequencies of interest. In our example of the sloping high-frequency hearing loss described above, the unmasked, as well as masked, high-frequency thresholds, would really generated from hair cells in the low- to mid-frequency region of the cochlea!

The whole concept might be clarified if we consider what might happen when lesser amounts of TEN are used. Imagine someone with a 20 dB hearing loss for the low frequencies and an 80 dB hearing loss for the high frequencies. Naturally, it would be at the high frequencies where cochlear dead regions might be suspected. Instead of immediately delivering 85 dB TEN, so as to just mask the high-frequency thresholds, let's deliver enough broadband TEN so that the good low-frequency thresholds are masked, for example, 50 dB of TEN. Here we should see the 20 dB low-frequency thresholds shifted to the 50 dB level of the TEN; however, the 80 dB thresholds for the high frequencies should not be shifted at all, because the TEN would not even be audible to the client at these frequencies. This would indicate a high-frequency hearing loss due to hair cells at the high frequencies that are damaged, but not completely dead.

On the other hand, let's suppose the high-frequency hair cells in this case are completely dead. Here, the broadband TEN presented at 50 dB might just have the effect of shifting not only the low-frequency thresholds but also the high-frequency thresholds! It might do so because the high-frequency thresholds seen on the audiogram do not truly arise from hair cells representing high frequencies. In fact, they could originate from the healthy existing inner hair cells representing the lower frequencies. Masking the lower frequencies with sufficient intensity to raise those thresholds thus would affect the thresholds at the higher frequencies where theoretically the TEN should not even be audible! Moore (2001), in his original article on cochlear dead spots, shows two examples of high-frequency hearing loss (with normal low frequency hearing), where various levels of TEN were presented. In one example, sufficient TEN to shift the better low-frequency thresholds has no effect on the higher-frequency thresholds where it normally should not be audible. In the other example, the same amount of TEN does indeed shift the higher-frequency thresholds. The only explanation for the second example can be the fact that the high-frequency thresholds are spurious and that they do not in fact arise from hair cells representing the high frequencies at all.

HEARING LOSSES COMMONLY ASSOCIATED WITH COCHLEAR DEAD REGIONS

At this point it may be useful to examine how the TEN test assesses two types of SNHL commonly associated with cochlear dead regions: the moderate rising or reverse hearing loss (Figure 2–2), and the severe precipitous high-frequency hearing loss (Figure 2–3). For either type of SNHL, the worst thresholds might very well be spurious; inner hair cells in these frequency regions might be dead, and the thresholds here could arise indirectly from healthier hair cell regions where the hearing shows better thresholds.

The TEN Test and Moderate Reverse SNHL

Be suspicious of immediately believing moderate reverse SNHL to be truly "moderate"; it could actually be indicative of a profound low-frequency SNHL, or dead inner hair cells in the low-frequency regions of the cochlea. Due to the

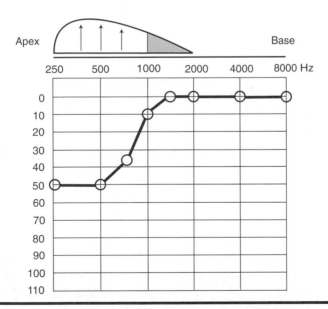

FIGURE 2–2   Low-frequency dead spots may reveal only a moderate, low-frequency SNHL with a reverse audiogram. Due to the long "tail" of the traveling wave, intense, low-frequency stimulation may "excite" the healthy mid-frequency hair cell regions (gray area). The person will indicate a response, but it will not truly arise from low-frequency hair cell regions. Note: Both steeply or gently rising reverse audiograms can be associated with low frequency cochlear dead regions.

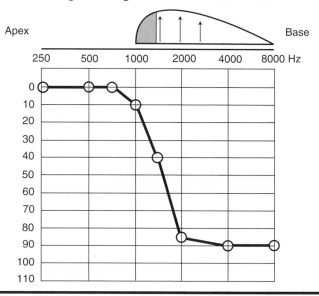

Severe Precipitous SNHL; Hearing Through Remote Hair Cells?

FIGURE 2–3   High-frequency dead spots may reveal an audiogram showing a precipitous, pronounced degree of high-frequency SNHL. Due to the steep "front" of the traveling wave, intense, high-frequency stimulation may "excite" the healthy mid-frequency hair cell regions (gray area). The person will indicate a response, but it will not truly arise from high-Hz hair cell regions. Note: Only steeply dropping thresholds can be associated with high frequency cochlear dead regions.

asymmetric shape of the traveling wave, however, only a moderate reverse hearing loss is revealed (Figure 2–2)! In other words, complete deafness in the low frequencies could masquerade as a moderate reverse SNHL. Here, it is important to realize that the steeply sloped front of the traveling wave faces the apex or low-frequency region of the cochlea, and the longer shallow "tail" slopes toward the base or high-frequency region of the cochlea.

Consider someone who has completely dead inner and outer hair cells for all of the low frequencies below 1000 Hz. Now imagine a 250 or 500 Hz tone presented from the audiometer, so that the peak of the traveling wave occurs in the dead low-frequency hair cell region at the apex of the cochlea. The dead low-frequency hair cells cannot respond, but the long shallow tail of the wave that extends into the mid-frequency region of the basilar membrane, can still stimulate the healthy mid-frequency hair cells. Even though the low-frequency hair cells might be totally dead, the moderate amount of low-frequency stimulation will still excite living mid-frequency hair cells, thus causing the person to raise a hand, indicating he/she indeed heard a tone (Halpin, Thornton, & Hasso, 1994)!

In this case, the person might be "hearing" these low frequencies with their healthy mid Hz hair cells, and not by means of their dead low-frequency hair cells. In some reverse SNHL, a relatively gentle rise in hearing thresholds as seen on the audiogram, is really a mirror reflection of the longer, more shallowly sloped "tail" of the traveling wave!

With cochlear dead regions of hair cells, one actually hears by means of remote, living hair cells. This is sometimes called "off-frequency hearing" (Moore, 2001). According to Moore's (2001) specific instructions and criteria, sufficient TEN should be presented in order to just mask the thresholds of interest—those at the lower frequencies where cochlear dead hair cells would be suspected—and then see whether the low-frequency thresholds were shifted by 10 dB or more above the TEN level. Here, however, the TEN might end up being presented at an intensity level enough to cause some loudness discomfort to the listener. An alternative is to present a small amount of ipsilaterally presented broadband TEN masking noise sufficient to make the good mid-to high-frequency thresholds worse. This would only be expected. If the reverse or precipitous high-frequency HL were due to cochlear dead spots, the TEN would, however, *also* elevate the thresholds for the worst thresholds, even though the TEN would theoretically be inaudible to the person at these frequencies!

Of course, not all reverse SNHL is due to cochlear dead spots. It is indeed very possible that the person could have a true reverse SNHL that is due to, for example, Meniere's disease. For that matter, one could also simply have a true hereditary moderate degree of low-frequency SNHL! If this were the case, a TEN level sufficient to mask the low-frequency thresholds would not shift the low-frequency thresholds by 10 dB more than the intensity of the TEN. Alternatively, if the TEN were presented at a softer intensity level so as to shift only the better mid- to high-frequency thresholds, little or no effect would be seen on the poorer low-frequency thresholds. Therefore, we might want to test whether the low-frequency hearing loss is really due to cochlear dead regions at the apex of the cochlea or not.

The TEN Test and Severe, Precipitous High-Frequency SNHL

Severe precipitous high-Hz SNHL can also indicate high-frequency cochlear dead regions (Figure 2–3). Here, it is possible that the high-frequency thresholds do not truly arise from damaged high-frequency hair cells; on the contrary, the high-frequency thresholds might result from indirect stimulation of low-frequency hair cells. The high-frequency hearing loss has to be severe because high-frequency stimulation would have to be quite intense to enable the steep front of the traveling wave to extend into the living, healthy mid-frequency hair cell regions. In the case of severe precipitous high-frequency SNHL, the steep slope of the precipitous high-frequency HL reflects the steep front of the traveling wave as it occurs in the cochlea!

Consistent with the direction shown in Figure 2–2, the steep slope of the traveling wave front faces the apex of the cochlea where the mid- to low-frequency hair cells are located (Figure 2–3). In this example, however, it is these low-to-mid frequency hair cells that are living. With intense high-frequency stimulation, the steep traveling wave front will spread just a bit into those living mid-frequency hair cells. Those hair cells will respond to the high-frequency tone, and the person will raise his/her hand saying the tone was heard. In this case then, even though the high-frequency hair cells might be totally dead, an intense high-frequency tone might stimulate mid-frequency hair cells. Since lots of intensity is required to accomplish this spreading of the traveling wave front, severe-profound high-frequency thresholds will be recorded on the audiogram. The severe-profound high-frequency thresholds are then not truly indicative of high-frequency sensitivity; rather, they occur as an artifact, a result of indirect stimulation of remote living hair cell regions. Again, since the front of the traveling wave is relatively steep, the behavioral thresholds will drop precipitously with progressively higher frequencies. The precipitous drop in thresholds, as seen on the audiogram, is really a mirror reflection of the steep front of the traveling wave!

In the case of the *precipitous high-frequency SNHL*, TEN could be presented at an intensity sufficient to just mask the poor high-frequency thresholds; the clinician would determine if the TEN caused the high-frequency thresholds to shift by an amount at least 10 dB above the intensity of the TEN itself. Alternatively, in order to reduce loudness discomfort, a lesser amount of TEN could be presented, just enough to shift the relatively good low-frequency thresholds. If the inner hair cells were truly dead at the high-frequency region of the cochlea, the TEN sufficient to mask the better low-frequency thresholds might also make the high-frequency thresholds worse, even though the same high-frequency thresholds were greater than the intensity of the masking noise! In all actuality, this would not seem possible, because these thresholds should not even be able to *hear* the masking noise. The reason why these thresholds would be affected, however, is because when one has dead hair cell regions at any frequency, one hears tones in these dead areas by means of a small piece of the traveling wave that extends into living hair cell regions.

The "Cookie-bite" SNHL

This relatively rare hearing loss configuration is often a genetic hereditary type of hearing loss, and these can also be due to mid-frequency cochlear dead spots. The cookie-bite SNHL presents with a moderate to moderately severe SNHL for the mid-frequencies, along with better low- and high-frequency thresholds. For a combination of reasons given earlier for reverse and for precipitous high-frequency SNHL, the moderate degree of mid-frequency thresholds can actually indicate cochlear dead spots in the mid-frequencies. In other words, normal low- and high-frequency hearing, along with total deafness in the mid-frequencies, can masquerades as a moderate (say, 50–60 dB) drop in mid-frequency thresholds; namely, a cookie bite SNHL.

THE TEN TEST: OLD VERSION IN dB SPL VERSUS AUDIOMETRIC TESTING IN dB HL

Up until very recently (Moore, et al., 2004), the TEN test with its pure tones and broadband masking noise were all calibrated in dB SPL, not HL. In this older version, the pure tones include octave and mid-octave frequencies from 125 to 10,000 Hz. Of course, the TEN is also broad enough in bandwidth to span this entire frequency range. In his earlier research, Moore (2001) also plotted subject results on audiograms where decibels were shown in terms of SPL. The TEN spectrum was specifically designed so that when it was ipsilaterally presented to normal-hearing subjects, it would yield flat, equal increases in thresholds across the frequencies. For example, TEN presented at 30 dB SPL would yield flat, 30 dB SPL hearing thresholds; TEN at 50 dB SPL would result in flat 50 dB SPL thresholds.

It is important to note the calibration in terms of dB SPL when attempting to use the older version of the CD in typical, clinical situations. Normal hearing thresholds tested from the TEN CD will not show a flat configuration when displayed on the typical audiogram, because the audiogram shows decibels in terms of HL. When plotting results of normal hearing straight on to the audiogram, the best thresholds generally appear for the mid-frequencies, with borderline to mild hearing loss for the low and high frequencies. Normal hearing is most sensitive to frequencies between 1 and 4 kHz, and this is best seen in terms of dB SPL. This is also the reason why equalizer buttons on some stereo systems are positioned to look like a "smile"; for softly presented sounds, we need the artificial boost for the lows and highs in order to hear all the frequencies equally loud. So also, for soft music on a stereo, we often push the "loudness" or "bass boost" button. With increases to overall intensity, we hear all frequencies equally loud, and thus, we no longer need the "loudness" or "bass boost," button activated. As with the upwards spread of masking, this is another well-known psychoacoustic phenomenon (Yost, 2000).

Accurately translating the TEN test results in dB SPL to the typical audiogram in dB HL requires some complicated calibration issues. This is a major consideration—and some would say, a clinical limitation—with the older TEN test version. To transform TEN test results from dB SPL into dB HL, various versions methods have appeared at different research and clinical centers where the CD has been used. The specifics, however, are beyond the scope of this introductory article, so I won't get into them here (besides, I hardly understand them myself). Unfortunately, at the time of the writing of this chapter, the case study results described in this chapter are those from the older TEN CD, calibrated in dB SPL. A newer version of the TEN test CD has recently been released, and it is calibrated in dB HL (Moore, et al., 2004). The specifics—and its availability—are described at the end of this chapter.

Case Studies with the TEN Test

The cases shown in this chapter were tested without any transforms between dB SPL and HL. The results from the TEN CD, calibrated in dB SPL, are simply plotted directly on to the audiograms. Still, the case study results here may be instructive in understanding the rational behind the TEN test.

CASE 1   **A Subject with Normal Hearing**

With the TEN presented at 30 dB SPL and the audiogram plotted in terms of dB HL, the hearing thresholds do not yield a flat configuration. As is actually shown in Figure 2–4, the unmasked thresholds from the normal-hearing subject appear best for the mid frequencies, worse for the lower frequencies, and worse also at 8000 Hz. When the TEN is presented to the same subject at an intensity of 30 dB SPL, the better thresholds are shifted more than the worst thresholds. One can assume that the thresholds that were shifted by the TEN were those where the TEN was audible, and that those thresholds that show no change are those where the TEN was not audible.

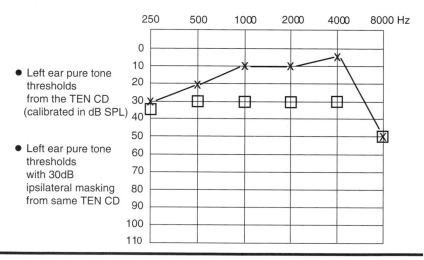

FIGURE 2–4   Hearing thresholds from the pure tones of the TEN CD were obtained from the author who has normal hearing in dB HL. Note that the thresholds from the pure tones of the TEN CD show a convex configuration. This is due to the calibration of the CD tones in dB SPL, whereas the audiogram is measured in terms of dB HL. Note also that the thresholds are masked by 30 dB TEN are only those thresholds that can hear it, and not, for example, the worst threshold at 8000 Hz.

CASE 2   A Subject with Sloping High-Frequency SNHL

Once again, the pure-tone thresholds in quiet show a slight hearing loss at 250 Hz; again, this is presumably due to the calibration of the CD in dB SPL (Figure 2–5). In this case, the TEN from the CD was presented at only 30 dB SPL, enough to mask the low-frequency thresholds but not enough to mask the high-frequency thresholds. Recall that this level is not strictly in accordance with Moore's (2001) instructions; namely, to present sufficient TEN to just mask the thresholds of interest—those at the higher frequencies where cochlear dead hair cells would be suspected—and determine if the higher-frequency thresholds were shifted 10 dB or more above the intensity level of the TEN itself. If this had been done for the present subject, the TEN would need to be presented much higher, at an intensity level enough to mask the thresholds at 4000 or 8000 Hz. Some subjects have reported excessive subjective loudness discomfort with TEN presented at levels of 60 or 70 dB SPL. In clinical situations, the TEN is thus sometimes presented at a level sufficient to mask the better hearing thresholds; at this intensity it is determined whether any effect upon the worse thresholds is observed. For this subject, with a TEN presentation of only 30 dB SPL, a shift does occur for the low-frequency thresholds, but a shift does not occur for the high-frequency thresholds. This would appear to make sense, because the subject here was not even able to hear the broadband TEN in the high frequencies. It would be assumed that this subject simply has high-frequency SNHL, but no cochlear dead regions.

Subject 2. Mild-Moderate SNHL
Cochlear Dead Spots Not Suspected

- Pure tone thresholds from TED CD (calibrated in dB SPL)
- Masked symbols: same CD, thresholds with 30B ipsilateral TEN

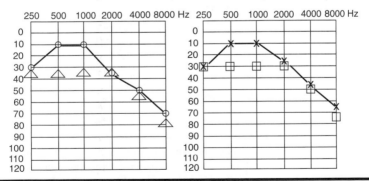

FIGURE 2–5 The ipsilateral masking with 30 dB TEN affects the better low-mid-frequency thresholds of the sloping SNHL, because the TEN is audible to the person at these frequencies. The TEN does not, however, affect the high-frequency thresholds because it is not audible to the person at these frequencies. This would indicate a typical high-frequency SNHL that is due to damaged hair cells at these frequencies, but not due to high-frequency cochlear dead spots.

A Subject with a Severe-Profound Mid-High-Frequency SNHL

The results are shown in Figure 2–6. As was done with the previous two subjects, thresholds for the pure tones from the TEN CD were obtained first, followed by thresholds found with ipsilateral TEN. Again, although the TEN level is much softer than that theoretically required according to Moore (2001), TEN levels that would mask the severe-profound mid-high-frequency thresholds would cause loudness comfort. As such, the subject's thresholds in quiet were compared to those in TEN presented at 50 dB SPL. If the mid-high-frequency thresholds truly arise from damaged (but not dead) hair cells regions representing those frequencies, the TEN at 50dB SPL would mask—and thereby shift—the low-frequency thresholds, but it would not have any effect on the high-frequency thresholds. However, as Figure 2–6 shows, the high-frequency thresholds are indeed affected with TEN at 50 dB SPL! This finding, says Moore (2001) would indicate cochlear dead spots for the high frequencies.

Subject 3. Severe Precipitous High-Hz SNHL Cochlear Dead Spots Would Be Suspected

- Pure tone thresholds from TEN Cd (calibrated in dB SPL)
- Masked symbols: same CD, thresholds with 50B ipsilateral TEN

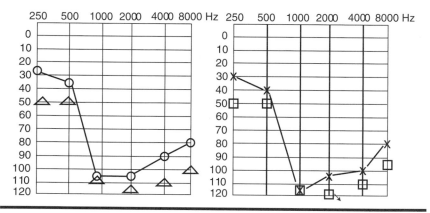

FIGURE 2–6   The ipsilateral masking with 50 dB TEN affects the low-mid-frequency thresholds of the sloping SNHL, because the TEN is audible to the person at these frequencies. The TEN also, however, shifts the high-frequency thresholds by at least 10 dB, even though it should not be audible to the person at these frequencies! This would be consistent with a high-frequency SNHL that is due to high-frequency cochlear dead spots. The high-frequency thresholds thus do not truly arise from damaged high-frequency hair cells; rather, they are a result of stimulation of remote hair cells at the low- to mid-frequencies that are responding to intense high-frequency stimulation ("off-Hz hearing").

DEAD REGIONS AND IMPLICATIONS
FOR AMPLIFICATION

For clients suspected of presenting with cochlear dead regions, amplification for their very worst thresholds might not be the best clinical course of action, because it would only provide useless information that would not benefit the client (Venema & McSpaden, 2004). In the case of reverse hearing loss (Figure 2–2), the low-frequency gain can result in irritability due to increased background noise. On the other hand, excessive high-frequency gain can result in annoying feedback for the person with precipitous hearing loss (Figure 2–3). The implications for amplification and cochlear dead regions are important; namely, don't focus amplification on the very worst thresholds. It might be best in these cases to amplify the transition of the audiogram; specifically, concentrate on those frequencies where the thresholds change in degree, not on where they bottom out or plateau at their very worst. For the reverse SNHL, this would involve the gentle (or more steep rise) of the audiogram; for the precipitous SNHL, the transition would be the steep slope itself.

Cochlear dead regions present unique challenges for hearing aid fittings because they often involve dramatic drops or rises between adjacent audiometric frequencies. Today's hearing aid technology, however, has increased in complexity at an exponential rate over the past 15 years, since approximately 1990. Multi-channel hearing aids, whether analog or digital, have independently adjustable channels, which enable an almost exquisitely accurate sculpting around the "corner" in an audiogram configuration. Even the analog two-channel hearing aids from the mid-1990s can do well here. For hearing losses that abruptly change at one frequency, it is important to have at *least* two channels, where one can provide very little gain/output, while the other can be turned up. The frequency crossover, where the two channels "meet," should be adjusted to be right at the "corner" of the audiogram, where the hearing thresholds begin to drop off. Much more is discussed about multi-channel hearing aids in Chapter 6.

Fitting a low-frequency rising (or reverse) hearing loss has indeed always been a challenge, especially for the older single-channel analog hearing aids of the past. Again, having two or more channels in a hearing aid allows for a much more accurate fitting in these cases. The fact that these reverse hearing losses can sometime be due to cochlear dead spots in the low-frequency region (apex) of the cochlea, however, can actually help to shed some light here! If the client reports that the low-frequency tones from an audiometer sound good and tonal in quality, the person may simply have a low-frequency hearing loss, and it may be a good idea to proceed with amplification. If this is the chosen strategy, then set the frequency crossover between the channels of the hearing aid so that it occurs at the "corner" of the audiogram, or where the hearing levels change. If the slope is gradual, then set the crossover frequency in the center of the rising slope. If, however, the client reports the low-frequency tones to sound "scratchy" or not very good in quality, then amplification might not be advisable for the worst low-frequency hearing thresholds. As such, it would not be surprising if the client with the reverse SNHL is not at all satisfied with their hearing amplification. Fitting the transition of the reverse SNHL or the rise itself might still be possible, however, because in this frequency region the hair cells are not completely dead.

For severe, precipitous high-frequency SNHL that is determined to result from cochlear dead regions, we would use the same kind of technology as we would to fit any other steeply dropping hearing loss, for example NIHL. The challenges are the same; namely, how do you fit the severe high-frequency thresholds without at the same time providing too much gain and output for the good hearing thresholds in the lower frequencies? Again, today's multi-channel hearing aids can provide a really good start. Set the crossover frequency between the channels so that it occurs at the "corner" of the audiogram, right where the hearing loss begins to plummet. Another thing to consider is just how much gain and output one should provide to the severe high-frequency thresholds. Recall that these thresholds may not be real at all, because the high-frequency hair cells are dead. Instead of providing most gain and output to the worst thresholds here, one may want to amplify with less gain and focus on the *transition* in the hearing loss; that is, amplify the slope of the hearing loss, not where it "bottoms out." This may sound contrary to one's intuition, but consider the alternative; amplifying at frequencies where there are no hair cells at all, and risking the client's intense dissatisfaction with useless high-frequency gain and excessive feedback.

Fitting the cookie-bite configuration of hearing loss is even more tricky, because now at least *three* channels are required—one for the low frequencies, one for the mid frequencies, and one for the high frequencies. In a three-channel hearing aid, there would likely be two frequency crossovers: one between the low- and mid-frequency channels, and the other between the mid- and high-frequency channels. If the cookie-bite SNHL dropped and suddenly improved, making it look like there were two corners in the audiogram, the two frequency crossovers could be set at the frequencies where the "corners" on the audiogram appear. If the slopes dropped and rose gradually, the crossover frequencies could be adjusted to occur around the centers of each of the two slopes.

PERCEPTIONS OF SOUNDS WITHIN A DEAD HAIR CELL REGION

For anyone with cochlear dead regions, one can only wonder what these sounds must "sound" like to the person. Perhaps it is a good question to ask, isn't it? If the person reports that the high-frequency tones don't really sound like tones at all, amplification for these worst high-frequency thresholds may not be such a good idea. If you see a person with a steeply dropping audiogram and severe-profound high-frequency thresholds, suspect high-frequency cochlear dead spots, and remember: You can help the dying but you cannot help the dead.

With cochlear dead spots, one hears tones in the dead areas by means of living hair cells in other cochlear regions. One can only wonder what this "off-frequency hearing" must sound like for the client! Some people report that these tones do not sound natural or tonal in quality. They sometimes report that pure-tone stimulation in these regions gives them a perception of a scratch or a tickle. These subjective reports, however, are not always consistent from person to person, even though dead areas might be indicated (Moore, 2001).

The author's recalls his clinical audiometry training, when he tested someone with a history of NIHL, who presented with a severe-profound high-frequency SNHL. A portable audiometer sat on a table, between the client and the clinician. A 4000 Hz pure tone was presented to the client under circumaural headphones at 90 dB HL. The client did not raise his hand, although the tone was audible to the clinician! When verbally asked if he could indeed not hear that tone, the client said, "I can feel it, but can't hear any tone."

Later on, in audiological practice, the author also recalls testing someone with a reverse SNHL. In this case, the client reliably raised her hand for the thresholds of near to normal hearing, namely, for pure tones at and above 1000 Hz. For the low-frequency tones (e.g., 250 and 500 Hz) however, the same client sometimes raised her hand at intensities as low as 40 dB HL, and sometimes as high as 60 dB HL. Her reliability was, hence, much poorer for her lower-frequency thresholds than for her higher-frequency thresholds. These findings today would have caused suspicion of dead low-frequency hair cells regions. First, the reverse SNHL configuration should cause some suspicion of cochlear dead spots. Second, the poorer reliability for her behavioral low-frequency thresholds may have resulted from off-frequency hearing, where the low-frequency stimuli were actually picked up from remote hair cells representing the high frequencies. From the position of hindsight (being 20/20), the author can only regret *not* having asked the client what those low-frequency tones actually sounded like.

A NEW VERSION OF THE TEN TEST

A newer version of the TEN test CD has been released, and it is calibrated in dB HL (Moore, et al., 2004). The pure-tone frequencies are more restricted than the older version; the new version includes octave frequencies only between 500 and 4000 Hz. The bandwidth of the TEN has also been reduced to encompass this narrower band of frequencies. The main advantage of the new TEN test calibrated in dB HL is that results can be translated accurately and transferred directly and to the audiogram without any need for transforming dB SPL values into dB HL. This also saves valuable clinical time, because the behavioral pure-tone thresholds only need to be tested once, not twice, as with the older CD calibrated in dB SPL. Furthermore, frequencies of clinical interest do not normally include assessment from 125 to 10,000 Hz, as found on the older version of the TEN CD. The more restricted pure-tone frequencies offered on the new CD also allow for a TEN with a narrower bandwidth. Thus, for any TEN level, the total noise intensity and loudness are reduced. In other words, since the very low and very high frequencies are eliminated, the overall intensity level of the TEN is reduced. As a result, the newer TEN CD no longer "pushes the envelope" of the audiometer output limits. Reduced overall intensity also reduces excessive subjective loudness discomfort on the part of the client (and the potential for causing NIHL while doing the test).

SUMMARY

- The TEN test on the CD is not, in the author's opinion, a required part of any new test battery for testing clients suspected of having cochlear dead regions. In fact, some research actually questions its clinical effectiveness and how well and consistently it identifies cochlear dead spots. Summers, Molis, Musch, Walden, Surr & Cord (2003) have shown that the TEN test sometimes renders false-positive indications of cochlear dead hair cell regions when for the same subjects, the gold standard behavioral test that would show the presence of dead cochlear hair cell regions (psycho-physical tuning curves) does not. As mentioned at the outset of this chapter, the knowledge required to understand the rationale behind the TEN test should be part of our education; understanding the TEN test for cochlear dead spots requires an appreciation for the fascinating way in which our cochleas work. This, in and of itself, far outweighs the necessity of obtaining the CD.

- The reverse, the severe, precipitous high frequency, and the cookie-bite SNHL should make the clinician suspicious that cochlear dead spots might exist. Most audiologists and hearing instrument specialists have encountered clients with these types of audiograms before; the concepts described in this chapter are intended to explain some of the underlying reasons *why* these audiograms are commonly associated with cochlear dead regions.

- It is a good idea to ask these clients about their subjective perceptions of audible tones presented to their worst thresholds; in other words, what do sounds in the dead regions actually sound like?

- These two small items—(1) initial suspicion and (2) secondary subjective questions—may really help when considering how much amplification to provide for a client's poorest thresholds. Should one concentrate on providing maximal low-frequency gain and output for the worst thresholds of someone's reverse hearing loss? For precipitous high-frequency SNHL, should one focus on amplifying the worst high-frequency thresholds?

REVIEW QUESTIONS

1. Outer hair cells provide about ____ / ____ dB gain for low and high frequencies, respectively.
    a. 10 / 20
    b. 30 / 40
    c. 50 / 60
    d. 70 / 80

2. In a rounded off number, how long in millimeters is the human "unrolled" cochlea?

   a. 35

   b. 45

   c. 55

   d. 75

3. According to Moore (2001), the TEN should initially be presented at an intensity that is sufficient to:

   a. just mask the best hearing thresholds.

   b. just mask the worst hearing thresholds.

   c. mask a threshold between the best and worst thresholds.

   d. none of the above

4. The original TEN test was calibrated in dB ____; the newer version is calibrated in dB ____.

   a. SPL / HL

   b. HL / SPL

   c. SL / HL

   d. HL / SL

5. A ____reverse SNHL should make the clinician suspect cochlear dead regions.

   a. mild

   b. moderate

   c. severe

   d. profound

6. A ____high-frequency SNHL could make the clinician suspect cochlear dead regions.

   a. mild

   b. moderate

   c. severe

   d. profound

7. Moore's positive criterion for the existence of cochlear dead regions is when the masked thresholds are:

   a. at least 10 dB above the TEN level.

   b. equal to the TEN level.

   c. 2 to 3 dB above the TEN level.

   d. actually below the TEN level.

8. The steep slope of high-frequency SNHL associated with cochlear dead regions arises from the:

   a. shallow front of the traveling wave.

   b. shallow tail of the traveling wave.

   c. steep tail of the traveling wave.

   d. steep front of the traveling wave.

9. The older version of TEN includes octave and mid-octave tones from:

   a. 125 to 8000 Hz.

   b. 125 to 10,000 Hz.

   c. 125 to 4000 Hz.

   d. 500 to 4000 Hz.

10. The new version of TEN includes octave and mid-octave tones from:

   a. 125 to 8000 Hz.

   b. 125 to 10,000 Hz.

   c. 125 to 4000 Hz.

   d. 500 to 4000 Hz.

ADDITIONAL RESOURCE

Where to get the new TEN Test CD (include mailing address where CD should be sent)

http://hearing.psychol.cam.ac.uk

25 US dollars, including shipping; payable to BCJ Moore

Prof Brian CJ Moore

Department of Experimental Psychology

University of Cambridge

Downing Street

Cambridge CB2 3EB

England

ACKNOWLEDGEMENT

The content of this chapter borrows heavily from two earlier articles that appeared separately in *The Hearing Professional,* which is the bi-monthly published journal of the International Hearing Society, Livonia Michigan:

REFERENCES

Halpin, Thornton, & Hasso. (1994). Low-frequency sensorineural hearing loss: Clinical evaluation and implications for hearing aid fitting. *Ear and Hearing, 15*(1): 71–81.

Moore, B. C. J. (2001). Dead regions in the cochlea: Diagnosis, perceptual consequences, and implications for the fitting of hearing aids. *Trends in Amplification 5*(1): 1–34.

Moore, B. C. J., Glasburg, B. R., and Stone, M. A. (2004). New version of the TEN test with calibrations in dB HL. *Ear and Hearing, 25*(5): 478–487.

Summers, V., Molis, M. R., Musch, H., Walden, B. E., Surr, R. K., and Cord, M. T. (2003). Identifying dead regions in the cochlea: Psychophysical tuning curves and tone detection in threshold-equalizing noise. *Ear and Hearing, 24*(2): 133–142.

Venema, T. H., (2003). Identifying cochlear dead spots. The Hearing Professional, July-August: pp 15–20.

Venema, T. H., and McSpaden, J. B. (2004). Cochlear dead spots: The fitting zone. The Hearing Professional, March-April, pp 19–22.

Yost, W. A. (2000). *Fundamentals of hearing: An introduction* (4th ed.). San Diego: Academic Press, Inc.

3

Why So Many Different Hearing Aid Fitting Methods?

INTRODUCTION

Hearing aid fitting methods are used to determine how much amplification to provide for clients having specific hearing losses. But for any specific hearing loss, there are many hearing aid fitting methods that can be used, and each one will lead to a prescription of somewhat different amounts of amplification at different frequencies. The student of hearing aids is often puzzled as to why so many different methods are used to fit hearing aids. The seasoned hearing health care professional may also wonder about the same thing. Each year, fitting methods, their rationales, and their respective updates are presented at conferences. Older fitting methods of the 1940s, all the way through the 1980s, were largely based on *linear* hearing aid amplification that dominated the scene, even as late as the late 1980s. These fitting methods were sometimes referred to as "threshold – based" fitting methods because they relied on the numerical value of the client's hearing thresholds. In keeping with hearing aid technology, as is the focus of this book, we will refer to these older fitting methods as "linear – based" fitting methods from now on. These fitting methods – as well as linear hearing aids themselves, will be discussed in this chapter.

Newer fitting methods consistently address *compression* in hearing aids. These fitting methods have been called "suprathreshold – based" fitting methods because, although they also utilize the client's hearing thresholds, they also address what takes place above one's hearing thresholds, such as, restoring normal loudness growth to the impaired ear. These newer fitting methods – which we will call "compression – based" fitting methods, will be covered in Chapter 4.

In the hearing health care discipline we are exposed to constantly evolving fitting methods and also new technology. One thing is certain: Regarding hearing aids, the fitting method(s) one learns at school will not necessarily represent all of the methods practiced at any future time in the real world by most clinicians. Thus, clinicians are often overwhelmed by the necessity of the constant learning process.

LENSES FOR THE EYE VERSUS HEARING AIDS FOR THE EAR

Fitting hearing aids is very different from fitting eyeglasses or contact lenses. More specifically, fitting hearing aids for presbycusis is a very different thing from fitting lenses for presbyopia. Some answers as to why we use so many different hearing aid fitting methods can be found if we look to another health science: Optometry. Sometimes defining who we are not helps us to get a better idea of who we are.

The general public is well aware that eyeglasses work better for the eye than hearing aids do for the ear. For the optometrist and the client, the fitting of lenses is either done correctly or incorrectly. The repercussions of an improper fitting of lenses are usually headaches or blurred vision. If this is not rectified, the person simply cannot wear the lenses. People do not normally go to visual rehabilitation classes, nor do they routinely return to optometrists for further instruction to learn how to use their eyeglasses after the initial fitting. After the lenses are prescribed, the person simply chooses the color and style of glasses he or she wants and the story usually ends there.

The general public is also aware that most typical vision problems result from an improper focus of light on the retina, which is situated against the back of the eyeball. In the simplest terms, the retina does for the eye what the cochlear hair cells do for the ear. The retina changes light into electricity, because electricity is the language the brain understands. A refocusing of light on an intact retina with properly fitted lenses is similar to fitting a person with *conductive* hearing loss with hearing aids. For the client with poor vision, incoming light that does not focus correctly on the retina has to be properly conducted, or refocused, so it can get to where it should go. For the client with conductive hearing loss, sound simply has to be amplified or conducted so that it can get through the middle ear to where it has to go (i.e., the hair cells of the inner ear).

If Optometrists had the same job as Audiologists or Hearing Instrument Specialists, they would most often be seeing clients with scratched or damaged retinas (Figure 3–1). For Optometrists, however, this is the exception and not the rule. In these rare cases (e.g. macular degeneration), even the proper focus of light on the retina will not bring about "normal" vision. We need to appreciate that this *is* the situation for the clinician fitting hearing aids. Only for conductive hearing loss is the cochlea intact. For the most part, hearing aids are fit on people with sensorineural hearing loss (SNHL), where the hair cells of the cochlea are damaged. This makes the problem more difficult than simply amplifying sound for a conductive hearing loss.

The hair cells of the cochlea are the "retina" of the ear (see Figure 3–1). Because most hearing loss results from damage to this "retina" of hearing, the fitting of hearing aids is different from the fitting of lenses, and the benefits of hearing aids are not always quite so obvious, especially to those who wear them! If the benefits of hearing aids are not clear to the client or if the hearing aids are physically uncomfortable, then clients simply will not wear them.

Fitting the Eye versus Fitting the Ear

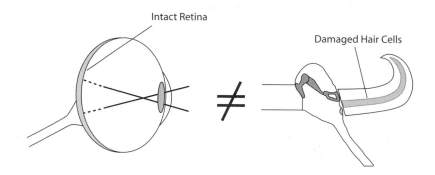

Intact Retina

Damaged Hair Cells

Hair Cells of the Cochlea are the "Retina" of the Ear

FIGURE 3–1   Optometrists and opticians refocus light toward the intact end-organ of the eye, the retina. In our field, audiologists and hearing instrument specialists must fit a damaged end-organ of hearing itself, namely the hair cells of the cochlea. The "retina" of the ear is the hair cells within the scala media of the cochlea.

The Audibility Problem

Since by far the most of hearing losses requiring hearing aids is SNHL, Hearing aids make incoming sounds louder, so persons with hearing loss can hear them. Persons with mild hearing losses are fit with low-gain hearing aids, and those with severe hearing losses are fit with high-gain hearing aids; persons with high-frequency hearing losses are generally fit with high-frequency emphasis hearing aids, and those with low-frequency hearing losses are generally fit with low-frequency emphasis hearing aids. This can be considered addressing the *audibility* needs of the client. Another big step towards addressing the audibility problem is to imitate the function of the outer hair cells with non-linear (compression) hearing aids, by deliberately increasing cochlear sensitivity to soft sound inputs below 40 to 50 dB SPL. This commonly achieved with a type of compression called "wide dynamic range compression (WDRC)." More on this will be discussed in Chapter 5. But beyond these considerations, what are the implications for clients if hearing aids are prescribed with one fitting method versus another? Will they get headaches? Will they really hear "better" when fit with one fitting method versus another? Here we reach the great impasse of hearing aid fitting methods: Choosing a fitting method is really a matter of choice, based on one's fitting philosophy, and not clearly a matter of correct versus incorrect.

When immersed in the clinical fitting of hearing aids, clinicians sometimes get bogged down by the absorption of new information. Think about what we are doing when we fit hearing aids. First, consider that, unlike the eyeball which is situated on the front of the face, the cochlea is buried almost an inch "behind" the outer ear or pinna. With the output sound from the hearing aids, we are smashing the eardrum with increased pressure and driving the middle ear ossicles harder than they were ever really meant to be driven, in the hope that the increased sound pressure will somehow increase the amplitude of the traveling wave and excite remaining undamaged hair cells in the cochlea. "Normal" cochlear function is certainly not restored with hearing aids; if it was, hearing aid fittings would be far more successful and fitting methods would be far fewer in number. It is truly interesting that no one hearing aid fitting method has been proven to be the "best" for any listening condition, let alone for speech intelligibility in background noise.

The Speech-in-Noise Problem

Increasing audibility is only half of the equation; increasing understanding of speech in background noise is the other part. Among modern-day humans, hearing is mostly a communicative sense we use to receive speech. Therefore, in the big picture of hearing and hearing aids, speech figures front and center. Vision, however, is mostly an environmental sense we use to negotiate and find our way in the physical world. Here it must be said that for the deaf community, vision and language share a special relationship because vision is the primary mode of receiving sign language. Deaf people use their eyes in more capacities than most hearing people could imagine. Witness the experience necessary to test persons with severe and profound hearing loss; they might raise a hand to a pure-tone presentation just because they see the examiner's shoulder move when the audiometer interrupter button is pushed.

For most people with hearing loss who wear hearing aids, hearing is the primary sense they employ to receive speech. For this population, increasing audibility is not enough; the added importance of *speech understanding in noise* cannot be overestimated. For students of hearing loss and hearing aids, this problem may not be self-evident or easy to comprehend. After all, those with typical hearing have problems hearing speech when there is a lot of background noise, but we get over it by yelling louder. Why is this then such a problem for those who wear hearing aids? If hearing aids amplify the speech and the background noise together, then why are people with hearing aids not in the same position as those with normal hearing? Why do those with hearing aids often complain bitterly about understanding speech in noise?

It's all about hair cells. The traveling wave cannot be sharpened with hearing aids, at least not at this time. As described in Chapter 1, damage to the outer hair cells results in a mild-to-moderate SNHL of around 50 dB HL; the damage also results in a broadened traveling wave, without the active sharpening that is normally provided by the outer hair cells. This may in turn result in poorer frequency discrimination and resolution for the client (Willott, 1991). However, provided that the hearing aids do not distort too much, a person with such hair cell damage may still do fairly well when listening to speech in background noise (Killion, 1997b). Again, as discussed in Chapter 1, outer hair cell damage often precedes damage to the inner hair cells.

Damage to the inner hair cells, however, has an even more dramatic effect on the ability to understand speech in background noise, because this results in a loss of afferent sound information to the brain from the cochlea. Persons with such damage lose the ability to separate or extract the speech from the background noise, and they need an abnormally large ratio of speech intensity relative to noise intensity, or an improved signal-to-noise ratio (SNR) to understand speech in noise (Killion, 1997b). If the speech and noise in some listening situation are equal in intensity, this is a 0 dB SNR. If the speech is 5 dB less intense than the noise, this is a -5 dB SNR; a + 5dB SNR occurs if the speech is 5 dB more intense than the noise.

According to Killion (1997a, 1997b) and Killion, Schulein, Christensen, Fabry, Revit, Niquette, & Chung (1998), to understand 50% of speech, speech has to be at least as intense as background noise, or there must be at least a 0dB SNR. Of course, the actual SNR required will depend on the specific type of speech stimuli used (monosyllables, spondees, sentences, etc.,) as well as the particular type of competing noise. For the sake of simplicity here, let's just say that for some particular experimental situation, normal hearing people would require a 0 dB SNR to understand 50% of the speech stimuli. According to the above-mentioned authors, those with a moderate degree of SNHL will require an *additional* 5 or 6 dB of speech in relation to background noise (a 5 – 6 dB SNR) to understand 50% of the speech. Therefore, in addition to requiring an increased audibility with their hearing aids, those with a moderate degree of SNHL will *also* require an additional 5 – 6 dB SNR when compared to normal hearing people.

These authors go on to state that each increase of 1 dB of speech relative to the background noise level will result in about a 10% improvement in speech intelligibility. Even if this number were to cut in half, such that each 1 dB increase of speech relative to background noise resulted in 5% improvement in speech intelligibility, these results would be quite remarkable. It is evident that quite a dramatic improvement in speech understanding can occur when the SNR is increased by only a few decibels. In a pitch to promote the usage of directional microphones, Killion (1997a, 1997b) and Killion, et al. (1998) suggest that directional microphones do indeed accomplish this increase in SNR by several dB. Much more will be discussed on directional microphones and their clinical benefits in Chapter 8.

Speech is meant to be understood, but all of its flowing, changing elements must be discerned as separate from aided background noise. Given the combination of (1) the nature of cochlear hair cell damage and (2) the present hearing aid technology, this goal is not readily achieved. If one cannot do well when listening to speech in background noise, even when aided with the best available technology, the best thing hearing aids can do in this case is to not cause any further problems (Killion, 1997b).

As we will see In Chapters 7 and 8, even the best or most promising of our digital noise reduction, cannot effectively subtract or *remove* background noise from the desired speech. When digital algorithms try to actually subtract background noise from speech, they also take out tiny, valuable pieces of sounds, or speech cues that are necessary for accurately perceiving speech. Hearing aids cannot replace the incredible function of normal hearing; when they try to separate speech from background noise completely, they tend to "throw the baby out with the bath water."

To better understand why this is the case, we should look at the unique properties of speech. Improving speech understanding in noise is not as simple a matter as making a steady-state pure-tone audible amid environmental background noise or the hubbub or babble of surrounding speech. This can actually be done quite easily with present digital technology. Making *speech* audible amidst background noise, however, is another matter. The ongoing pops and fizzes of frontal, consonantal sounds, the combinations of tonal elements, and the temporary closures of our vocal tracts defy an easy characterization and an easy separation from background noise, even with the assistance of mathematical algorithms used in current digital hearing aids (see Chapter 7). Speech consists of complicated acoustic signals that are rapidly changing in intensity and frequency over time.

In a rather humorous experiment (Bentler & Duve, 1997), an 1880s speaking tube was tested against two popular digital hearing aids on the Auditec Speech in Noise™ test at a cocktail party. The background noise levels were a moderate 83 dB SPL. The results were about equal for all three "contestants." This finding suggests that we have not yet solved the problem of removing background noise from speech, even with digital hearing aids.

In summary, given these realities, it is no wonder that fitting hearing aids for ears has not been as exact a science as fitting lenses for eyes. Unlike the case for Optometry, in our field, it is usually the "retina" of the ear that is affected. Furthermore, aside from an inability to sharpen the traveling wave, the target of amplification is speech, which is often spoken when there is also surrounding background noise. Without hearing aids, people with hair cell damage hear soft, garbled speech that is difficult for them to separate from the background noise; with our present-day hearing aids they hear louder speech and noise. For hearing aids today, separating speech from background noise is easier said than done. *Audibility* of speech may be improved, but *clarity* of speech is not necessarily improved with hearing aids, especially in the presence of background noise. Clinicians – and hearing aid technology – have traditionally dealt with audibility. It seems, however, that our hearing impaired clients themselves had the job of teaching us, the clinicians, about the speech-in-noise problem. We are slowly learning; today, we have basically two basic methods of dealing with the difficulties of listening to speech in background noise. One of these is the directional microphone. When used on hearing aids, it is well known to slightly improve the SNR. The other method is digital noise reduction, which has not consistently been shown to improve the SNR. Again, much more will be discussed on each of these methods in Chapter 8.

For now, we should take a look at a short history of hearing aid technology, so we can appreciate the distance we have come, especially over the past 15 years. Following this, we will look at the evolution of fitting methods. It is important to look at these developments in this order, because fitting methods evolved out of a fusion or compromise between two things: 1) the knowledge that with SNHL, one's sensitivity for soft sounds is reduced, although one's loudness perception for intense sounds is similar to that for normal hearing, 2) the available linear hearing aid technology of the day.

A SHORT HISTORY OF HEARING AID TECHNOLOGY

In the first half of the 20th century, hearing aids had a remarkably limited frequency response and, therefore, were fit mostly on persons with flat conductive hearing losses or gently sloping SNHL. Most were "body" style hearing aids that had a flat frequency response that dropped off above 2000 Hz. Individuals with flat hearing losses could be fit with these hearing aids, but clients with steeply sloping high-frequency SNHL, often called "tractor deafness," were told nothing could aid this type of hearing loss. Choosing a hearing aid for a particular client was a simple matter of deciding whether he or she needed one.

Around 1900, hearing aids were carbon based, which means the microphone was filled with carbon granules (Hodgson, 1986). Incoming sound pressure made patterns in the resistance of the carbon granules, which resulted in patterns of electrical current that were then transduced back into sound by a magnetic "earphone," or receiver. The microphone and receiver had to have overlapping resonances and so the carbon hearing aids had a narrow frequency response with a single peak.

The 1920s saw the development of vacuum tube hearing aids that were much more powerful than carbon-based hearing aids, but also quite large and inflexible in frequency response. The earlier ones had crystal microphones, which were much more efficient than the carbon microphones. Vacuum tube hearing aids required *two* batteries: one to heat the filaments inside the vacuum tubes and another to provide the general power for amplification. Due to their large size, these vacuum tube hearing aids could not be worn on the ear.

In the 1950s the transistor replaced the vacuum tube and hearing aids became much smaller with better high-frequency emphasis (Hodgson, 1986). Because transistors were so much smaller than vacuum tubes, they required far less power and, thus, the battery size became smaller. Frequency responses also became more flexible and could provide anything from a broad- or wide-frequency response to more high-frequency emphasis. Over the past two decades, the typically sharp peaks in the frequency responses and the distortion seen in earlier hearing aids have been reduced. Interestingly, even though hearing aid distortion has been reduced, as late as the 1970s it was sometimes still so bad that even people with *normal* hearing had problems when they wore hearing aids and listened to speech in background noise (Killion, 1997b).

Advances in Hearing Aids

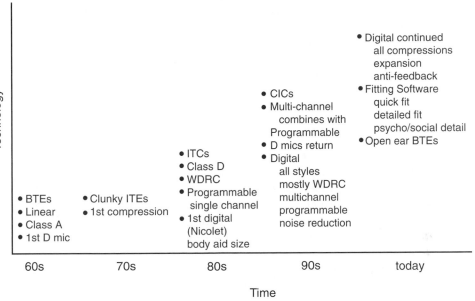

FIGURE 3–2 The development of hearing aids continued slowly up until the 1990s. Then, a dramatic upturn of events in hearing aid technology took place. Perhaps coincidentally, it is also at this time that the distinct role of the outer hair cells found its way into field of clinical practice.

Body-style hearing aids gave way to behind-the-ear (BTE) hearing aid styles in the late 1950s, and these soon became the norm. The BTE style also became incorporated in a hearing aid–eyeglass combination. This may have had some cosmetic appeal, but the hearing problem remained when wearers took off their glasses, they also removed their hearing aids.

In the 1960s, in-the-ear (ITE) styles began to appear (Figure 3–2). The first ITEs were modular, which meant that they snapped onto a custom-made ear mold. Later developments led to nonmodular ITEs, with circuits built into ear mold shells. Cosmetic desires by consumers for hearing aids that were least visible drove the manufacturing industry to emphasize the production of ITEs. In the early 1980s, smaller canal hearing aids began to appear, and in the 1990s, the even smaller completely-in-canal (CIC) styles became ever more popular. The big advantage of CICs was to reduce the occlusion effect, as the receiver end of the hearing aid was to be in contact with the boney portion of the ear canal. In all reality, however, the endeavor has not always been readily achieved, because of the physical discomfort that often accompanied these tight fittings.

In the present decade, it appears that the BTE is coming back; but this time, a few changes are evident. First, the actual size of the BTE housing has become even smaller. Next, much thinner tubing connects the ear hook of the BTE to the generic ear bud inserted into the ear canal. These new BTEs are often called "open fit" hearing aids, because the typical vented ear mold used with conventional BTEs, is replaced with a generic ear bud that has many holes in it. It is simply selected from a finite set of different sizes to best accommodate the ear canal of the client. This amply vented ear bud dramatically reduces the occlusion effect; hence, the name "open-fit." In essence, the open-fit BTE combines BTE feature of housing the hearing aid electronics safely away from the cerumen of the ear canal, along with the improved cosmetics of the CIC. The first open-fit BTEs (Avance™ and later, the Air™) were introduced by ReSound in 2000 and 2003, respectively. Realizing the potential for fitting success with this style, many other manufacturers followed suit in 2004 and 2005. For a good discussion on styles of hearing aids, the occlusion effect, and much more, the reader is encouraged to read the textbook called *Hearing Instrument Technology,* by Vonlanthen (2006). The reader is also encouraged to read Martin (2005) for a short, concise summary on the values of the new open-fit, thin-tubed BTEs.

Another major development in hearing aids has been the types of circuits that have become available; namely, the nonlinear or, "compression," hearing aid circuits. Prior to the 1970s, analog linear circuits in hearing aids prevailed; some persisted to the mid 1990s. Most of these had class A or B amplifiers (see Appendix A). Already beginning in the early 1970s, nonlinear or compression hearing aid circuits began to augment manufacturer offerings of linear hearing aid circuitry. The first compression hearing aid circuit was produced in 1972 by Linear Technology (now Gennum) in Burlington, Ontario Canada. Class D amplifiers, associated with much longer battery life, appeared in the 1980s. By the mid 1990s, compression circuitry became the norm. At first, compression was offered as an output limiting solution for those who experienced loudness discomfort. In the early 1990s, WDRC emerged as a type of compression that provides greatest gain for soft input sounds, so as to mimic the role of the OHCs.

In 1987, Nicolet produced the world's first digital hearing aid (called the Phoenix™) but due to its body-aid style size, it did not gain acceptance. In 1996, the first digital technology appeared in BTE and ITE styles. This was the Senso™, produced by Widex. Digital technology is able to combine linear, output limiting compression, WDRC, and much more, into a single package. In general, hearing aid technology really took off around 1990 (Figure 3–2). Slow, steady growth prevailed over the decades until the 1980s; hearing aid development after that seems to have taken an exponential turn (Figure 3–2). Much more concerning compression and digital technology and also the events of the 1990s and today, as outlined in Figure 3–2, will be described further in later chapters.

Linear Hearing Aids

For now, the concept of "linear" needs to be elaborated, because it is the *interaction* between linear circuitry in hearing aids and the exquisitely nonlinear cochlea that gave rise to the vast array of fitting methods that arose during the

Linear Amplification

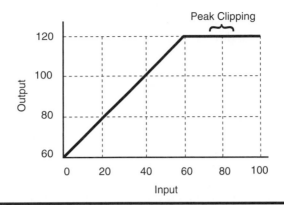

FIGURE 3–3   With linear hearing aids, the output increases correspondingly along with the input. In this example, the gain of the linear hearing aid (shown by the 45° line) for various input intensity levels, is 60 dB. For example, for 20 dB inputs, the output is 80 dB; for 60 dB inputs, the output is 120 dB; for 100 dB inputs, the output would theoretically be 160 dB (if not for output limiting)! Normal hearing people - and those with SNHL - usually cannot tolerate much more than about 120 dB SPL. Linear hearing aids limited the maximum power output with "peak clipping" (shown as the 180° horizontal line at the 120 dB SPL output). In this case, any output more than 120 dB SPL would be clipped or "cut off."

latter half of the last century. Those original fitting methods have also formed the basis of today's compression-based fitting methods (covered in Chapter 4).

The first hearing aid fitting methods were based on or assumed the use of linear circuitry in hearing aids. To understand linear hearing aids, it is important to be familiar with the most basic formula for hearing aids: Input + Gain = Output (see Figure 3-3). "Input" is whatever sound enters a hearing aid, "gain" is the amount of amplification given to the input by the hearing aid, and "output" is the sum total of sound that travels from the hearing aid and into one's ear.

An output intensity of 120 dB sound pressure level (SPL) is usually uncomfortably loud for both those with normal hearing and individuals with sensorineural hearing loss (SNHL). Normal conversational speech averages at about 65-70 dB SPL. If a hearing aid supplies 45 dB of gain to, say, 70 dB, then its output approaches 120 dB SPL. For a person with a similar uncomfortable listening level, this may be the maximum gain we can add to the intensity of average, on-going speech before the discomfort level is reached. As long as the input sounds are about 70 dB or less, the output sounds from the hearing aid will remain below the uncomfortable listening level for that person. If the input level rises above 70 dB, then the added gain of 45 dB will result in an output that exceeds 120 dB SPL, and the person will have discomfort.

A hearing aid that provides the same amount of gain for any and all input intensity levels is known to provide linear gain (Figure 3–3). That is, the aid produces 1 dB of output for each decibel of input (a 1:1 ratio) up to a certain maximum output limit. For example, if a hearing aid has 50 dB of linear gain at full-on volume, then it will provide 50 dB of gain to 10 dB SPL input sounds as well as to 70 dB SPL inputs. The corresponding outputs will be 60 dB SPL and 120 dB SPL, respectively. The first output would be tolerable for most individuals, but the second probably would not. When hearing aid outputs exceed a wearer's uncomfortable listening level, the remedy of linear circuitry is to "clip the peaks" of the maximum output. This was usually accomplished, by means of peak clipping, with a maximum power output (MPO) control on the hearing aid.

The main problem with limiting the output with peak clipping is that when the output sound exceeds the set MPO, the hearing aid becomes saturated and distorts the sound and the *quality* of listening is sacrificed. If a hearing aid provides 60 dB of gain and the MPO is set to around 120 dB SPL, then the typical speech inputs of 70 dB SPL will constantly drive the hearing aid into saturation; and this will result in poor sound quality. When the peaks are clipped, the receiver diaphragm (like the cone of a speaker) is literally restricted in its back-and-forth movements. When this happens, sine waves of sounds are literally turned into square waves, which are complex sounds. In short, simple sinusoids containing single frequencies are converted into complex sounds containing more than one frequency. This is how harmonic distortion is produced. Linear hearing aids were the "state of the art" in hearing aid technology until the mid 1970s and even in the 1980s, most hearing aid fittings involved linear circuitry.

In summary, linear hearing aids are called "linear" because they provided the same gain for all input sound levels. On an input-output graph (Figure 3–3), the line showing the function of linear hearing aids is straight or linear (until the maximum power output is limited and peak clipping occurs). Compression hearing aids, on the other hand, provide *different* amounts of gain for different input sound levels. There are many different types of compression hearing aids and for any one of these, the line on an input-output graph showing the function of a compression hearing aid is not straight. Hence, compression hearing aids are often called nonlinear hearing aids. More is discussed about input-output graphs and also the wide topic of compression in Chapter 5.

A SHORT HISTORY OF LINEAR – BASED FITTING METHODS

Fitting methods themselves only address audibility. They do not specifically address the SNR required for the hearing impaired to hear better in background noise. In any fitting method, mathematically determined amounts of amplification (or gain) are derived from the client's numerical thresholds at specific frequencies, according to some specific formula.

As discussed earlier, outer hair cell damage, resulting in the most common type of cochlear hair cell damage, results in a mild-to-moderate degree of SNHL.

What has not been specifically addressed regarding those with SNHL is the issue of loudness tolerance for intense sounds. More will be discussed on this topic in Chapter 4.At this point, it is sufficient to note that for most people with SNHL, the "ceiling" of loudness tolerance for intense sounds does not change significantly; it is the "floor," or the ability to hear soft sounds, that changes most.The loss of hearing sensitivity thus changes mainly at the soft end of the hearing range; thus, SNHL does *not* result in a need to have all sounds amplified by the *same* amount. On the contrary, they require soft sounds to be given the most amplification, and loud sounds to be given little or no amplification.

Therefore, the first hearing aid fitting methods arose out of a compromise between (1) the knowledge that for SNHL, sensitivity for soft sounds is reduced, although the loudness perception for intense sounds is not, and (2) the available linear hearing aid technology at the time, which amplified soft and intense sounds by the same amount.

Hearing aid fitting methods have evolved over the past half century as a result of a mixture of hearing aid technology available at any particular time and the experimental trials and errors of scientific inquiry. Carhart (1946) developed a clinical comparative approach of trying several hearing aids on the same person to determine the "best" one for speech recognition and which one the person "liked" the best. His approach involved various speech test measures in unaided and aided conditions with each of several different hearing aids. Typically at that time, clinicians relied on their own internal criteria, which were often based on personal experience with particular hearing aid models. It soon became clear that it was difficult to teach this method to someone else and to generalize the criteria from one clinic to another. Clinicians began to feel the need for a systematic *prescription* approach to fitting hearing aids, a system that could be followed by anyone anywhere.

Can't We Just "Mirror" the Audiogram with Gain?

"Mirroring" the audiogram would simply imply providing as much gain as the hearing loss itself. If a person's hearing loss is 20 dB HL for the low frequencies and 50 dB HL for the high frequencies, a mirror reflection of this hearing loss would then imply providing 20 dB of gain for the lows and 50 dB of gain for the highs. This would theoretically take all sounds below one's hearing threshold and reposition them so they are above one's hearing thresholds.At first glance, this approach of amplifying by the amount of hearing loss itself might seem like the intuitive thing to do. If attempted, however, it would soon become clear that we cannot simply "mirror" the audiogram with this amount of gain, at least not with linear hearing aid amplification.

Figure 3–4 (left panel) shows an audiogram with a pronounced high-frequency hearing loss.The right panel of Figure 3–4 shows the same audiogram flipped upside-down, so the concept of mirroring the audiogram might become clearer. If it were possible simply to amplify incoming sound by the degree of the hearing loss, then there would be only one fitting method needed. Clinicians would fit hearing aids "correctly" or "incorrectly," and new fitting methods would

"Mirror" the Audiogram with Full Gain?

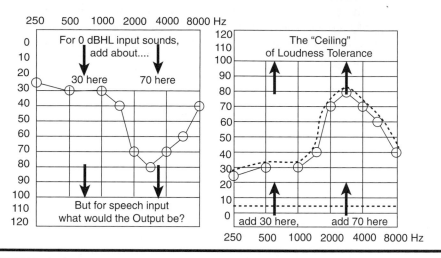

FIGURE 3–4 "Mirroring" the audiogram with amplification seems like the intuitive thing to do. But if this were true, there would be only one fitting method! The left panel shows the typical audiogram as obtained in most clinics. The right panel shows intensity now read as "up," similar to the way we read hearing aid specifications sheets. The dotted lines show 5 dB HL sounds that could be amplified so they are audible to the person. But could speech inputs be amplified by the same amount?

not surface every year. To students learning about hearing aids and to practicing clinicians this would be a relief. Alas, this is not our reality. Let's look at this more closely.

"Mirroring" the audiogram seems intuitively correct because we could make all thresholds "0" for the person's hearing loss. That is, 0 dB HL input sounds would then become "just barely audible," much like they are for persons with "perfect" hearing. Slightly more intense sounds, like 10 dB HL, would become audible at a sensation level of 10 dB, and so on. But what about more intense sound inputs, like speech? Can we amplify all sounds equally? Again, not with linear hearing aids.

"Mirroring" the audiogram with full linear gain could only be closer to the truth, if the tolerance for loudness grew along with the hearing loss, as it would with an earplug stuck in the ear—or for conductive hearing loss. In this case, both thresholds and loudness tolerance would be elevated and we could simply overcome the increased impedance with amplification. If all we had to do was deliver the "lost dBs" to an intact cochlea, then we could simply match the hearing aid gain to the degree of hearing loss. For, example, a 60 dB hearing loss would be fit with a 60 dB gain hearing aid.

Most people with hearing loss, however, have SNHL with the *dynamic range* smaller than normal. Dynamic range is the "area" of residual hearing between the hearing thresholds (softest levels one can hear) and the uncomfortable listening levels (loudest levels one can tolerate). Consider the example of someone with mild hearing loss in the low frequencies and moderate hearing loss in the high frequencies, who has uncomfortable loudness levels of, say, 100 dB HL at all audiometric frequencies. For this person, the dynamic range, the area between thresholds and loudness tolerance levels, would be smaller for the high frequencies than for the low frequencies.

Most people with SNHL have a reduced dynamic range, where soft sounds are not audible, and yet, intense sounds are still heard as loudly as they are by those with normal hearing. The "floor" of hearing sensitivity is elevated, but the "ceiling" of loudness tolerance is relatively unchanged. Hearing aids for someone with this type of loss must amplify soft sounds below the person's threshold by a lot; but intense sounds cannot be amplified by the same amount without dramatically exceeding the person's tolerance for loudness. More is discussed on dynamic range in Chapter 4.

Killion and Fikret-Pasa (1993) rejected the concept of "mirroring" the audiogram with full gain, but their reasons were different than those given here. They stated that mirroring the audiogram is unrealistic, because it would amplify background noise too much. Mirroring the audiogram of a person with a SNHL of 40 dB HL would mean giving a full 40 dB of gain for the person to hear 0 dB HL sounds. This would theoretically restore normal hearing, but the sound pressure level of most background ambient noise is about 40 to 45 dB(A). Even a person with normal hearing levels is not able to hear audiometric pure tones softer than 20 to 25 dB HL in this common environment. A full gain of 40 dB would amplify both the ambient 40 to 45 dB(A) of background noise and the 20 to 25 dB HL pure tones buried within it. Therefore, providing a full 40 dB of gain would be too much gain. Killion argued that a better gain target for the 40 dB sensorineural hearing loss would be less (e.g., around 20 to 25 dB).

Basically, we cannot use linear hearing aids that amplify various intensity levels of sound inputs by the same amount; if we do, we will have to choose hearing aids that offer less gain overall. This is exactly what Lybarger found by trial and error as early as the 1940s (Lybarger, 1944)!

Lybarger's Half-Gain Rule

Lybarger (1963) proposed a "half-gain" rule that seemed to work well with linear hearing aids, which were the "state of the art" of hearing aid technology at the time. When fitting people who had SNHL with full-gain hearing aids (e.g., 60 dB gain for a 60 dB HL input), he would talk to clients and ask them to turn the volume to where they liked it. They would usually turn the volume halfway up. Thus, by trial and error, Lybarger found that most people preferred about half the gain for their hearing loss (e.g., 30 dB gain for a 60 dB hearing loss). In this way, his clients could get a comfortable amount of gain for both soft and loud speech and still be able to tolerate the output. The half-gain rule is a *compromise* between (1) the linear circuitry he had available at the time and (2) the reduced dynamic range of the damaged nonlinear cochlea.

The half-gain fitting method is still in use today because it forms the basis of many subsequent "linear" fitting methods developed in the 1960s, 1970s, and 1980s. A few of the more popular "children" of the half-gain rule are: Berger's half-gain method (Berger, Hagberg, & Rane, 1979), prescription of gain and output (POGO) by McCandless and Lyregaard (1983), the one-third gain method by Libby (1986), and the National Acoustics Lab-revised (NAL-R) by Byrne and Dillon (1986).

Linear-based fitting methods offered an alternative to the requirements of the comparative methods of speech testing as outlined by Carhart (1946). The required gain for these methods is determined from the thresholds and is presented as a theoretical target. The actual gain from any hearing aid is matched to the target to determine how close it comes to meeting the goal. According to McCandless and Lyregaard (1983), speech intelligibility testing was time-consuming and showed a lot of statistical variability. On the other hand, a numerical approach (based on the client's hearing thresholds) with a specific gain target could more easily identify the required frequency response of hearing aids. The results of hearing aid trimmer settings and changes to these settings were also more visible with threshold-based fitting methods than they would be with tests of speech discrimination and speech reception in a sound field (Libby, 1988; McCandless & Lyregaard, 1983).

Typical half-gain linear-based fitting methods offer a single "target" of gain for any one particular hearing loss configuration, because they all assume linear hearing aid circuitry (which provides the same gain for all input levels until the output saturates). These methods assume that the target gain should be met with the volume control of the hearing aid set to a user setting. They also share the suggestion that the hearing aid should have about 10 to 15 dB extra or reserve gain above and beyond the user volume control setting (Libby, 1988). All the linear - based fitting methods discussed here attempt to maximize the intelligibility of speech at the client's most comfortable listening level. These fitting methods also include suggestions for determining the MPO of a hearing aid to prevent the aided gain from exceeding the client's uncomfortable loudness levels (UCL).

For most of these fitting methods, the gain prescribed for the lower frequencies is less than that prescribed for higher frequencies. This is done to reduce the "upward spread of masking" (see Chapter 1). One of the main complaints of hearing aid wearers is that of amplified background noise competing with amplified speech. Background noise consists of many frequencies. Colloquial clinical knowledge has it that the "hubbub" of background speech noise is mostly low-frequency energy, while the mid-to-high frequencies contribute more weight to the intelligibility of speech. Because low frequencies mask high frequencies better than highs mask lows, amplified background noise may indeed wreak havoc with speech intelligibility, especially for those who wear hearing aids.

It is interesting to note, however, that for any particular hearing loss, the targets suggested by these older fitting methods are all markedly different, as shown in Figure 3-5. Figure 3-5 is a rough sketch of four older linear - based

A Comparison of Threshold Methods

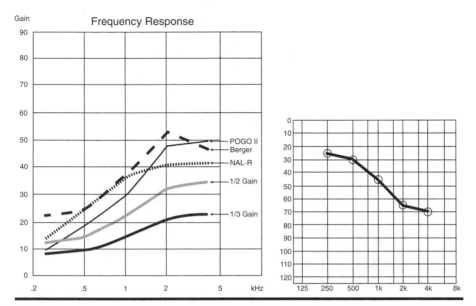

FIGURE 3–5   Five different linear – based fitting methods give five different targets for the same person's hearing loss! There is even one more complication; the differences between the targets, themselves, vary with different hearing losses!

fitting methods derived from the half-gain rule. All provide a single target based on the thresholds of the audiogram because all assume linear hearing aid gain. As such, all of these fitting methods are markedly out of date because almost all of today's hearing aids provide nonlinear (compression) gain. The methods are covered here mainly in the interest of providing a historical perspective.

The Berger half-gain fitting method surfaced earlier than the others. For the hearing loss in Figure 3–5, the Berger fitting method offers the most gain at 1000 and 2000 Hz. For this fitting method, the most important speech cues for optimal understanding were believed to be at these particular frequency regions. Therefore, more than one-half gain was offered for 1000 Hz and 2000 Hz. Less than one-half gain was offered for the low frequencies to optimize speech intelligibility and reduce the upward spread of masking. To arrive at the specific gain requirements for a particular hearing loss, Berger suggested the following: multiply the hearing loss at 250 Hz by .45, at 500 Hz by .50, at 1000 Hz by .625, at 2000 Hz by .667, at 3000 Hz by .588, at 4000 Hz by .50. These multiplication values represented the various weights of importance for speech intelligibility that Berger attached to each audiometric frequency. Berger recommended a reserve gain of 10 dB. To calculate maximum power output, Berger converted uncomfortable listening levels (measured in a sound field) to units of dB SPL, and then setting the MPO 4 to 6 dB above this level (Berger, Hagberg, & Rane, 1979).

The POGO method came into use after the Berger method (McCandless & Lyregaard, 1983). For the hearing loss in Figure 3–5, POGO asks for about as much high-frequency (4000 Hz) gain as Berger's method. The POGO method is quite straightforward in its calculations: It asks for exactly one-half gain at each audiometric frequency (multiply each threshold by .50), with less than one-half gain for the low frequencies of 250 Hz (10 dB less) and 500 Hz (5 dB less). The Berger and POGO fitting method give similar weight to the high frequencies, because these frequencies are thought to contribute greatly to speech intelligibility. However, POGO proposes considerably less gain for the mid and low frequencies than the Berger method, in order to further reduce the possibility of the upward spread of masking. Like the Berger method, a 10 dB reserve gain is also suggested by POGO. McCandless and Lyregaard (1983) note that a reason for some hearing aid rejections was that of exceeding uncomfortable loudness levels with the hearing aid gain requirements. Accordingly, the maximum power output is another parameter of concern for POGO. Unlike the Berger method, POGO suggests that the MPO on the hearing aid should be set to the client's UCL as measured in dB hearing level (HL).

The Libby one-third–two-thirds gain fitting method is similar to that of POGO, except that for those with mild-to-moderately severe hearing losses, the thresholds at each audiometric test frequency are multiplied by one third. According to Libby (1986), these clients and those with precipitous high-frequency hearing losses do not actually wear their hearing aids at a volume that provides one-half gain for their hearing losses. On the contrary, these clients tend to prefer a volume setting that reflects a gain closer to one third of their thresholds. Like the Berger and POGO methods, Libby suggests relatively less gain for the low frequencies of 250 Hz and 500 Hz. Perhaps because of the reduced overall gain suggested by the one-third gain method, Libby recommended a reduction of only 5 dB from one-third gain at 250 Hz and 3 dB from one-third gain at 500 Hz. For severe and profound hearing losses, Libby recommended a two-thirds gain rule, because he found these people to prefer more gain.

The NAL-R fitting method seems to have surfaced in popularity later than the other methods mentioned, and in the author's experience, it is the most popular of the linear-based fitting methods today. The main focus of NAL-R method is to amplify unaided adjacent speech frequencies so that they sound equally loud at a comfortable listening level, and thus maximize intelligibility of speech for people with hearing loss. The original NAL fitting method (Byrne & Tonnison, 1976) was subsequently found not to consistently accomplish this objective and so the NAL method was revised (Byrne & Dillon, 1986)—hence, the NAL-R fitting method. One figure in the article by Byrne and Dillon (1986) shows NAL and NAL-R targets superimposed on a fictitious flat audiogram of 0 dB HL, and reveals that the revised NAL provides about 10 dB more gain at 500 Hz, and about 3 to 4 dB more gain at 3000 and 4000 Hz than the original NAL. In general, NAL-R provides slightly less than half-gain across the audiometric frequencies. The target gain configuration of NAL-R usually looks "flatter" than those prescribed by most other linear fitting methods. Many audiologists believe NAL-R is "kind" to steep, high-frequency hearing losses because it prescribes less high-frequency gain than Berger or POGO. Perhaps the ability to reach NAL-R targets with available hearing aids psychologically added to its allure. At any rate, NAL-R remained for years the most popular method for fitting mild-to-moderate hearing losses in North America. Today compression-based fitting methods (to be discussed in Chapter 4) have by now taken over.

In general, for any particular hearing loss, NAL-R suggests slightly less than one-half gain. The NAL-R method also tries to prevent excessive high-frequency gain for clients with steeply sloping hearing losses. It requires a more complex calculation than the other mentioned fitting methods to determine the appropriate gain. The calculation has three elements: (1) a constant value, obtained from the average thresholds of 500 Hz, 1000 Hz, and 2000 Hz multiplied by .05; (2) thresholds at each audiometric frequency threshold are multiplied by .31; and (3) different gain values for each frequency required to make various frequency regions of speech sound equally loud. As to the third element in the NAL-R calculation, the low frequencies are given less gain than the mid frequencies (e.g., 117 dB for 250 Hz), and the high frequencies are given slightly less gain than the mid frequencies (e.g., 12 dB for 4000 Hz). These three elements must be added together to determine the prescribed gain for each audiometric frequency. For more explanation or specifics, the reader is encouraged to read the original NAL-R article by Byrne and Dillon (1986).

Figure 3–5 shows that the gain proposed by the NAL-R fitting method is less than POGO for the high frequencies and more than POGO for the low frequencies. Compared to Berger, the suggested gain for NAL-R is similar for 500 and 1000 Hz, but is less at 2000 Hz and higher. The NAL-R fitting method suggests a 15 dB reserve gain above the client's user volume control setting.

In Australia, a further development of NAL-R resulted in the NAL-RP (Bryne, Parkinson, & Newall, 1990). We haven't seen much of the NAL-RP here because it was incorporated into later versions of the NAL-R fitting method. The NAL-RP included some additional specific considerations for severe-to-profound hearing losses. First, it was noted that those whose audiometric pure-tone average (500, 1000, and 2000 Hz) is greater than 60 dB generally prefer about 10 dB more than half gain. Second, the authors discovered something very important and unexpected in people with sloping severe-to-profound hearing loss. If the hearing thresholds at 2000 Hz were 90 dB or more, those clients actually preferred *more* low-frequency gain and *less* high-frequency gain, than their counterparts who have a more flat hearing loss configuration! Hair cell regions where there is severe-to-profound hearing loss are so damaged that they do not have much to contribute to someone's hearing and speech recognition ability. The main implication here: amplify less at frequencies where there is severe-to-profound hearing loss, and amplify more at frequencies where there is better hearing. In the vernacular of the previous chapter on cochlear dead regions, the message could be, "You can help the dying but you cannot help the dead."

There is now a version of NAL, called the NAL-NL1 (which stands for Non-linear, version 1), which is based on compression hearing aids; this is discussed further in Chapter 4.

It should be reiterated that all of the linear-based fitting methods briefly described here provide a *single* target for any one particular audiometric hearing loss configuration, because they assume linear amplification (which provides the same gain for all input sound levels). Each method acknowledges that the most common type of hearing loss is sensorineural in nature, and, also, that although soft sounds are inaudible, intense sounds may still be heard as loud as they would for normal hearing. The result of this phenomenon is a reduced dynamic range. The target for any particular hearing loss and for any particular threshold-based fitting method arises out of a *compromise* between the reduced dynamic range encountered with SNHL and linear hearing aid technology.

SUMMARY

- Unlike optometry, there is no single, universally accepted hearing aid fitting method; that is, the fitting is not necessarily done "correctly" or "incorrectly."

- Simply "mirroring" the audiogram with full linear gain is impossible, because for those with SNHL, the "floor" of hearing sensitivity may be elevated compared to normal hearing, but their "ceiling" of loudness tolerance is similar to those with normal hearing. The half-gain method of Lybarger arose out of a compromise between (1) the linear technology available at the time and (2) the nonlinear function of the cochlea.

- Many of the older linear – based fitting methods were derived from the half-gain fitting method. These methods assume linear circuitry. They all focus on numerical values of audiometric thresholds, and acknowledge a reduced dynamic range with SNHL, but they do not focus specifically on loudness growth. Loudness growth and some newer compression – based fitting methods will be discussed in Chapter 4.

REVIEW QUESTIONS

1. If speech is presented at 50 dB HL and noise is 40 dB HL, this is a _____ dB signal-to-noise ratio (SNR):

    a. 0
    b. 10
    c. –10
    d. 90

2. Killion (1997a) says an increase in SNR by 1 dB results in a speech reception improvement of:
   a. 10%.
   b. 50%.
   c. 100%.
   d. none of the above

3. As pertains to hearing aid development, the 1950s was the decade of the:
   a. vacuum tube.
   b. carbon-based microphones and receivers.
   c. compression circuits.
   d. transistor.

4. Today's tiny BTEs with the very thin tube connecting to a stock ear mold are often called:
   a. thin air BTEs.
   b. open-fit BTEs.
   c. vented ear mold BTEs.
   d. none of the above

5. The very first directional microphones in hearing aids appeared around the:
   a. 1960s.
   b. 1970s.
   c. 1980s.
   d. 1990s.

6. A linear hearing aid provides 100 dB output with 40 dB input; the gain is:
   a. 140 dB.
   b. 60 dB.
   c. -60 dB.
   d. not enough information given here

7. The same linear hearing aid saturates at a 120 dB SPL output; what's the output with a 70 dB SPL input?
   a. 110 dB SPL
   b. 120 dB SPL
   c. 130 dB SPL
   d. 140 dB SPL

8. Which of the four fitting methods discussed in this chapter recommend most gain at 2000 Hz?

a. Berger

b. POGO

c. Libby

d. NAL-R

9. Which of the four fitting methods discussed in this chapter recommends the least amount of overall gain?

a. Berger

b. POGO

c. Libby

d. NAL-R

10. Which of the four fitting methods discussed in this chapter was by far the most popular?

a. Berger

b. POGO

c. Libby

d. NAL-R

RECOMMENDED READINGS

Byrne, D., & Dillon, H. (1986). The National Acoustics Laboratories' (NAL) new procedure for selecting gain and frequency response of a hearing aid. *Ear and Hearing, 7*(4): 257–265.

Killion, M. C. (1997). The SIN report: Circuits haven't solved the hearing-in-noise problem. *The Hearing Journal, 50*(10): 28–34.

Lybarger, S. F., & Lybarger, E. H. (2000). A historical overview. In R. Sandlin (Ed.), *Hearing aid amplification* (pp. 1–35). San Diego: Singular, Thomson Delmar, Inc.

McCandless, G. A. (1994). Overview and rationale of threshold-based hearing aid selection procedures. In M. Valente (Ed.), *Strategies for selecting and verifying hearing aid fittings* (pp. 1–18). New York: Thieme Medical Publishers, Inc.

Vonlanthen, A. (2006). *Hearing instrument technology.* Clifton Park, NY, Thomson Delmar Publishing

REFERENCES

Bentler, R. A., & Duve, M. (1997, April). *Progression of hearing aid benefit over the 20th century*. Poster session presented at American Academy of Audiology, Fort Lauderdale, FL.

Berger, K. W., Hagberg, E. N., & Rane, R. L. (1979). Determining hearing aid gain. *Hearing Instruments, 30*(4): 26-44.

Byrne, D., & Dillon, H. (1986). The National Acoustics Laboratories' (NAL) new procedure for selecting gain and frequency response of a hearing aid. *Ear and Hearing, 7*(4): 257-265.

Byrne, D., Parkinson, A., & Newall, P. (1990). Hearing aid gain and frequency response requirements for the severely/profoundly hearing impaired. *Ear and Hearing, 11*, 40-49.

Byrne, D., & Tonnison, W. (1976). Selecting the gain of hearing aids for persons with sensorineural hearing impairments. *Scandinavian Audiology, 5*, 51-59

Carhart, R. (1946). Tests for selection of hearing aids. *Laryngoscope, 56*, 780-794.

Hodgson, W. R. (1986). Hearing aid development and the role of audiology. In W. R. Hodgson (Ed.), *Hearing aid assessment and use in audiologic habilitation* (pp. 1-12). Baltimore: Williams and Wilkins.

Killion, M. C., & Fikret-Pasa, S. (1993). The 3 types of sensorineural hearing loss: Loudness and intelligibility considerations. *The Hearing Journal, 46*(11): 1-4.

Killion, M. C., (1997a). "I can hear what people say, but I can't understand them." *The Hearing Review, 4*(12): 8-14.

Killion, M. C. (1997b). The SIN report: Circuits haven't solved the hearing-in-noise problem. *The Hearing Journal, 50*(10): 28-34.

Killion, M. C., Schulein, R., Christensen, L., Fabry, D., Revit, L., Niquette, P., & Chung, K. (1998). Real-world performance of an ITE directional microphone. *The Hearing Journal, 51*(4): 24-38.

Libby, E. R. (1986). The 1/3-2/3 insertion gain hearing aid selection guide. *Hearing Instruments, 37*(3): 27-28.

Libby, E. R. (1988). Hearing aid selection strategies and probe tube measures. *Hearing Instruments, 39*(7): 10-15.

Lybarger, S. F. (1944). U.S. Patent Application SN 543, 278.

Lybarger, S. F. (1963). *Simplified fitting system for hearing aids.* Canonsburg, PA: Radio Ear Corp.

McCandless, G. A., & Lyregaard, P. E. (1983). Prescription of gain and output (POGO) for hearing aids. *Hearing Instruments, 34*(1): 16-21.

Willott, J. F. (1991). *Aging and the auditory system: Anatomy, physiology, and psychophysics.* San Diego: Singular Publishing Group, Inc.

4

Compression and the DSL and NAL-NL1 Fitting Methods

INTRODUCTION

In this chapter, the psychoacoustic concepts of normal versus abnormal loudness growth and also, two of the more popular newer hearing aid fitting methods are discussed. In contrast to the older methods discussed in Chapter 3, these methods assume the use of compression in hearing aids; furthermore, they focus not only on the client's hearing thresholds, but also on what takes place *above* the hearing thresholds, namely the "growth" of loudness. This is why they have sometimes been called "suprathreshold" fitting methods; in keeping with the terminology of Chapter 3, however, we will call these newer fitting methods "compression – based" fitting methods. Compression – based fitting methods emerged in the 1990s and have rapidly gained in popularity.

Loudness growth occurs from one's hearing thresholds, with perceptions of sounds ranging from "just barely audible" up to the loudest sounds that one can tolerate. The decibel "area" that lies between these two extremes, is called one's *"dynamic range."* Basically, a dynamic range can be calculated from the decibel level of one's loudness tolerance levels (for speech or for pure tones) minus that of one's speech reception threshold (SRT), or pure-tone thresholds. For the sake of simplicity, we will just refer to loudness tolerance level in the singular form.

A typical dynamic range for the mid frequencies is about 100 dB, where the thresholds are close to 0 dB HL and the loudness tolerance level is at around 100 dB. For people with this dynamic range, a 50 dB HL sound might be perceived as "comfortable" in loudness. For a mild-to-moderate sensorineural hearing loss (SNHL), such as presbycusis, however, a 50 dB HL sound might be barely audible, whereas the loudness tolerance level will still be at around 100 dB HL. In this case, the dynamic range is smaller (50 dB) and loudness "grows" much faster than it does for the normal-hearing person with the wider 100 dB dynamic range. Compared to someone with normal hearing, the "floor" of hearing sensitivity is elevated for the person with the SNHL; on the other hand, the "ceiling" of loudness tolerance is about the same as it is for someone with normal hearing.

Many clinicians want to restore normal loudness growth for their clients. There are sounds in our environment that those with normal hearing perceive as "soft," "comfortable," and "loud." Ideally, for persons with hearing loss who wear hearing aids, these sounds should be perceived the same way. If this objective is accomplished with hearing aids, then normal loudness growth has been restored for the client. In the example of the person with mild-to-moderate SNHL, restoring normal loudness growth may require a hearing aid that provides very different gain for soft input sounds (such as 20 dB HL) than it does for more intense input sounds (such as 80 dB HL). Only a *compression* hearing aid can accomplish this objective.

As discussed in Chapter 3, linear hearing aids provide the same gain for different input sound levels. Fitting methods that generate a single target of gain for a particular hearing loss assume linear amplification, because the target is applicable for any input sound level of intensity. However, the gain for *different* input levels is not specifically addressed by these methods. For example, since conversational speech is usually of the most interest, the gain targets of these older fitting methods is intended to place the loudness of the input sound (conversational speech) into the middle of the dynamic range of the listener. The idea here is to place amplified conversational speech at or near the most comfortable loudness of the listener. Unfortunately for the listener, however, the resultant gain with the linear hearing aid will be the same for a whisper as it will be for the loudness of conversational speech. In other words, conversational speech might be given sufficient amplification, but inputs like a whisper will not be given enough. So also, inputs that are louder than conversational speech may very well receive too much gain and will sound uncomfortably loud to the listener, or else cause the hearing aid to go into peak clipping or saturation.

Compression – based fitting methods provide more than one target, where each target represents a different amount of gain (or output) that is prescribed for specific, different intensities of input sound levels. These fitting methods specifically address compression because compression provides *different* amounts of gain (and/or output) for different input intensity levels. Two of the more popular of these fitting methods will be described further in his chapter: The Desired Sensation Level (DSL) fitting method, and the National Acoustics Laboratories nonlinear version 1 (NAL-NL1) fitting method. Both originate from vast British Commonwealth countries that usually appear as pink in color on a world globe. The Desired Sensation Level (DSL) method, developed at the University of Western Ontario in Canada, began with the interest of fitting infants, and it has its own unique considerations. The NAL-NL1 method, developed at the National Acoustic Labs in Sydney, Australia, evolved from the older linear-based NAL-R method, in order to specifically address compression.

Today's hearing aids almost exclusively use compression; linear hearing aids are now the exception. This ratio was the reverse only about 15 – 20 years ago. Many different types of compression are discussed specifically in Chapter 5. Some types of compression are especially effective at limiting the output to not exceed one's uncomfortable loudness level (UCL). On the other hand, there are some types of compression where the specific goal is to shrink a normal (large) dynamic range into a smaller range that occurs with SNHL. No one compression can be said to be "better" than another; the choice of compression for any particular case depends on the clinical objective and what type might be best for the client.

In this chapter, the concepts of loudness growth, new fitting methods, and the need for compression are discussed together. A reduced dynamic range and consequent abnormally rapid growth of loudness is the problem the person with hearing loss takes to the clinician. Compression-based fitting methods set up the ideal aided gain and output targets for the client. The various types of compression in hearing aids (discussed in Chapter 5) are the ways or means whereby to accomplish the goals that are set out by the fitting methods.

LOUDNESS GROWTH AND CONSEQUENCES OF A REDUCED DYNAMIC RANGE

As mentioned in Chapter 1, hearing aids cannot replace the internal function of the cochlea with its active traveling wave and mechanically mobile outer hair cells. But we are making small steps toward this goal. Figure 4–1 shows what present hearing aid technology *can* do to imitate the function of the outer hair cells for mild-to-moderate SNHL, namely, help restore normal loudness growth. Note in the figure, the horizontal axis represents the physical world of intensity and the vertical axis represents the corresponding psychoacoustic perception of loudness.

SNHL usually exhibits a reduced dynamic range. The normal-hearing person in Figure 4–1 has a dynamic range of 100 dB, which means that 0 dB HL sounds are perceived as "just barely audible" and 100 dB HL sounds are perceived as "too loud." For the hearing loss, the dynamic range is only 50 dB, because the threshold (for some particular frequency) is 50 dB HL and the uncomfortable loudness level is 100 dB HL. Note that 100 dB is perceived as "too loud" for both the normal-hearing person and the person with mild-to-moderate SNHL. The difference for the two populations is mainly for perception of low-intensity sounds. The loudness "growth" "just barely audible" to "too loud" is more rapid or steep for the person with the SNHL than it is for those with normal hearing. The "ceiling" of loudness tolerance is the same with both normal hearing and with SNHL, but the "floor" of hearing thresholds is elevated with the SNHL.

What should a hearing aid do in this situation to best imitate the function of the outer hair cells? It should restore normal loudness growth. In other words, soft inputs, when amplified, should sound "soft" to the listener who is wearing the hearing aid; medium inputs, when amplified, should sound "comfortable" to the same listener; and intense inputs should sound "loud." To accomplish the goal of restoring normal loudness growth with hearing aids, soft input sounds need to be amplified by a lot, and loud input sounds should be amplified by little or nothing at all. At high intensities, the role of the hearing aid should "disappear" or according to Killion (1997) it should become acoustically

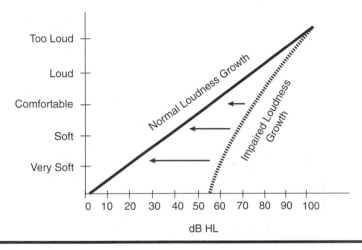

Loudness Growth:
Normal Hearing vs
Sensorineural Hearing Loss

FIGURE 4–1   The goal of amplification for mild-to-moderate SNHL is to restore normal loudness growth. The X axis shows the physical/acoustic dimension of increasing input sound intensity to the hearing aid. The Y axis shows the corresponding psychoacoustic dimension of increased loudness perception. We don't know how to sharpen a traveling wave with hearing aids yet. But we can amplify soft sounds more than loud sounds. To do this, a hearing aid should amplify soft sounds by a lot, and loud sounds by little or nothing at all.

"transparent." The cochlea is a nonlinear organ; just because thresholds increase does not mean that loudness tolerance levels increase as well. Accordingly, we should provide nonlinear gain with hearing aids so that low-intensity input sounds are amplified by more than high-intensity input sounds.

A word of caution should be noted regarding the commonly cited loudness growth graph shown in Figure 4–1. The reader is encouraged to read a very interesting article by Florentine (2003), which contradicts this typical loudness growth model. During the typical pure-tone threshold hearing test, clinicians may have noted that those with SNHL often give a quick behavioral response to audible tones where their thresholds are elevated. This might indicate that at frequencies where their hearing loss exists, sounds near their thresholds are not exactly perceived as "very soft." On the contrary, they may perceive instead a sudden indication of audible sound, which then rises rapidly in loudness as the intensity is increased towards their loudness tolerance levels (Florentine, 2003).

There is one thing missing from Figure 4–1, namely, frequency. Figure 4–2 includes the physical dimensions of frequency and intensity, along with the psychoacoustic dimension of loudness growth. The curves shown in Figure 4–2

With SNHL:
The "Ceiling" is the same, but the "Floor" is raised

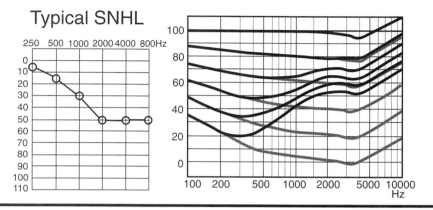

FIGURE 4–2   Frequency, intensity, and loudness growth are shown together in one graph. Note that intensity (vertical axis) shows decibels in terms of SPL. Normal hearing for one ear under a headphone is shown by the bottom curve. This bottom curve corresponds to 0dB HL on the typical audiogram. Here we can see that for mild-to-moderate SNHL (darker lines), the "ceiling" of loudness tolerance is the same as it is for normal hearing; it is the "floor" of hearing sensitivity that becomes elevated for the hearing loss. The cochlea is indeed a nonlinear organ.

are sometimes called "equal loudness contours," "Fletcher-Munsen curves," or "phon" curves. In addition, the loudness growth for normal hearing and for a typical mild-to-moderate SNHL is compared.

The lighter curves, or contours, show equal loudness perceptions for normal hearing across the frequency range. Along any one particular curve, each frequency along the bottom axis sounds equally loud to normal ears; note that each frequency requires a different SPL to be perceived as equally loud. This difference in required SPL is especially evident for the lower curves.

The bottom-most curve is closest to what is known as 0 dB hearing level (HL). Sometimes called the "minimal audibility curve," this bottom contour represents the perception of "just barely audible" by normal hearing listeners, with one ear under a headphone. It shows that our best hearing is somewhere between 1000 and 5000 Hz. To be just barely audible, the low frequencies and extreme high frequencies need to be more intense (in dB SPL) than the mid frequencies. At high intensities such as 100 dB SPL, however, the curves flatten out. In other words, for high intensities, there is less *difference* in SPL required for us to judge the sounds at all the frequencies as being equally loud. Here it becomes evident once again, that the cochlea is a nonlinear organ; that is, for equal loudness perceptions across the frequencies, the cochlea works differently with soft sound inputs than it does for intense sounds.

The shape of the bottom-most curves has a lot to do with why we have a "loudness" switch on our stereo or why on equalizers the buttons are often arranged like a "smile." At low-volume control settings, we need an extra boost for some frequencies to hear all the frequencies equally loud. At high-volume settings, however, the equal loudness lines flatten out. This means that for intense sounds we no longer need as great a difference in sound pressure levels across the frequency range to hear all the frequencies equally loud and this is why we then turn the loudness switch off.

For normal hearing, there is a normal spread of the curves or loudness contours. Note that the dynamic range, or area, between the top and bottom curves in Figure 4–2 is largest for the mid frequencies and smallest for the very low frequencies. A smaller dynamic range implies a "faster" loudness "growth." For example, the smaller dynamic range for the low frequencies means that the growth of loudness from sensations of "just barely audible" to "very loud" is relatively fast compared to that for the mid frequencies. The equal loudness contours for normal hearing show a dynamic range of about 100 dB near 1000 Hz.

For the SNHL (the darker curves in Figure 4–2), the top curves for are similar to those for normal hearing. On the other hand, the bottom curves become elevated for the mid to high frequencies. The curves that are squeezed, or pinched, together in the mid to high frequencies show a smaller dynamic range. For these high frequencies, the person with SNHL cannot hear soft sounds. Yet high-intensity sounds are perceived just as loudly as they are by people with normal hearing. Once again, for the person with normal hearing and the person with SNHL, the "ceiling" is the same; it is the "floor" that is elevated for the person with hearing loss. Loudness growth is more rapid for the high frequencies where the ceiling and the floor are closest together.

It could and perhaps should be asked as to why these curves exist in the first place. Why does the human minimal audibility curve (the bottom-most curve) show differences in hearing sensitivity in the first place? The difference in normal hearing sensitivity is largely caused by the physical properties of the middle ear and the outer ear (Yost, 2000). As a system of physical structures, the middle ear has its own sum total characteristic properties of mass and stiffness, and thus has its own resonances that pass some frequencies through more easily than others. As discussed briefly in Chapter 1, the middle ear is not as efficient at passing some frequencies as it is at others. The resonances of the concha (4000 to 5000 Hz) and outer ear canal (1500 to 4000 Hz, with a peak around 2700 Hz) also contribute to the shape of the human minimal audibility curve.

COMPRESSION AND NORMAL LOUDNESS GROWTH

Recall from Chapter 3 the basic hearing aid formula: *input* plus *gain* equals *output*. Linear hearing aids give the same gain for all input levels, and threshold-based fitting methods that assume linear amplification offer a single target for gain, which is based on the thresholds of the hearing loss. Because the gain is the same for all input intensity levels in linear circuits, there is no need for more than one target. For high-intensity input sounds, a linear hearing aid with a lot of gain will give an output that may exceed one's loudness tolerance levels and so the maximum output is "clipped," which may result in distorted sound quality.

Compression hearing aids do not limit the maximum output with peak clipping; rather, they use compression to accomplish this objective. What is compression? It is the provision of progressively less and less gain, for greater and greater input intensity levels. Compression is specifically described and explained in Chapter 5. For now, it is sufficient to understand that as one's dynamic range becomes smaller - and loudness growth consequently becomes more rapid - more compression is required.

For compression hearing aids, a single gain target no longer tells the whole story, because *compression circuits provide different amounts of gain for different input levels*. Compression tends to reduce the gain as the input levels increase; however, this should not be done at the expense of making the *outputs* all the same for these different input levels. The output for each input level is important to consider, because the output is the real result or "goods" that reaches the ear of the person wearing the hearing aid. If the gain does go down as much as the input levels go up, then the outputs for different levels of inputs will all sound equally loud, and the person wearing the hearing aid will not be able to tell when things are actually getting louder in the real world.

Most gain should be given to soft input sounds, so the person with SNHL can hear the sounds. Recall that for SNHL, the threshold "floor" is raised, while the loudness tolerance level "ceiling" is not. Gain should be provided so as to elevate soft sounds to reach the raised floor. For example, a person with a 60 decibel (dB) hearing loss trying to listen to 1 or 2 dB hearing level (HL) sounds should in theory be given 60 dB of gain. As the inputs increase in intensity, the gain should go down, but again, not quite as much as the amount by which the inputs increase. The outputs will then still increase with input level, but not by as much as the inputs increase. In this way, persons with hearing loss still experience a growth of loudness for sounds as they naturally occur in the environment. Thus, a normally large dynamic range will be "shrunk" into a smaller one (more on this topic will be covered in the section on WDRC, in Chapter 5).

Newer fitting methods that address compression hearing aids specify the desired gain and output for several input levels (e.g., soft, medium, and loud inputs). As clinicians, we often see advertisements for certain compression hearing aids where the stated goal is to "restore normal loudness growth" for the client who demonstrates "abnormal" loudness growth. Indeed, many nonlinear (or compression) hearing aids are specifically designed to "restore normal loudness growth" for the person who has SNHL and a smaller-than-normal dynamic range. We now come to the specific discussion of the two most popular compression-based fitting methods today: the DSL and the NAL-NL1 fitting methods. Each fitting method has a very different slant.

DSL FITTING METHOD

The Desired Sensation Level fitting method originated in 1982, and it was specifically intended to address the needs of the pediatric fitting population. The development of oral speech and language depends first and foremost on the *audibility* or ability to hear all of the sounds of speech. This is especially important for children who experience their hearing loss before or during speech and language acquisition. The DSL fitting method is an attempt to make the soft, medium, and loud sounds of speech audible and comfortable for such children. It has continued to develop and evolve as hearing aid technology advanced. For example, in 1991, DSL mainly concerned linear hearing aids, as most hearing aids being fit then were linear. Later on, DSL[i/o] was developed to address compression (Cornelisse, Seewald, & Jamieson, 1994). DSL may have began out of concern for the fitting requirements of the pediatric population, but its use has also been generalized to adults (Seewald, 1997). The fitting algorithm of DSL is still being constantly updated.

Figure 4–3 shows the spectrum of speech superimposed on an audiogram. The vowels have relatively more intensity and lower frequency content (i.e., louder and lower) compared to the unvoiced consonants, which have higher frequency content and less intensity (i.e., softer and higher). In the big picture of speech reception, the vowels tell us *that* we hear speech. Every word contains at least one vowel. Our discrimination of *what* word we hear, however, depends heavily on the audibility of vowel/consonant sound combinations.

To this end, the main goal of DSL is the *audibility* of speech. To make as much use of residual hearing as possible, the entire unaided speech spectrum must be amplified to fit above the hearing thresholds and yet below the loudness discomfort levels (i.e., within the dynamic range) of the person with hearing loss. Furthermore, the amplified speech spectrum must be as comfortable and undistorted as possible.

For the DSL fitting method, the input signal of conversational speech is represented by the unaided long-term average speech spectrum (LTASS). The LTASS measurements for DSL were derived using a microphone placed at the ear level of a child (Cornelisse, et al. 1994) rather than the customary placement of the microphone in front of a subject (Cox & Moore, 1988). As a result, the DSL group found that the LTASS consisted of relatively more low-frequency energy (close to 70 dB SPL) and less high-frequency energy than the measurements by Cox and Moore (1988). It is also important for children to hear their own voice production of high-frequency consonants to properly acquire speech (Cornelisse, Gagne, & Seewald, 1991). These measures of LTASS, together with the focus on audibility of all speech sounds, lend towards the observed fact that DSL provides more low and high frequency output than other fitting methods.

One thing that originally characterized DSL and set it apart from most other fitting methods, was its fitting graph—the SPL-o-gram. The audiogram, loudness tolerances, and the fitting targets for any specific client are all placed on this graph (Figure 4–4). As on the typical audiogram, the SPL-o-gram places frequency

Speech Sounds on an Audiogram

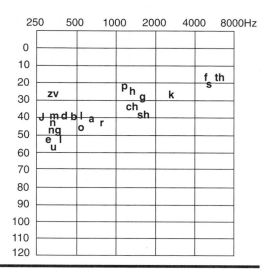

FIGURE 4–3 The slope of the energy present in speech rises from left to right on the typical audiogram. The vowels are more intense and lower in frequency compared to most consonants, especially the unvoiced consonants, such as /s/, /f/, /th/, etc. For someone with high frequency hearing loss, the unvoiced consonants will be especially hard to hear. Thus, the high frequency speech sounds will obviously need to be amplified the most to make them audible.

The "SPL-o-gram"

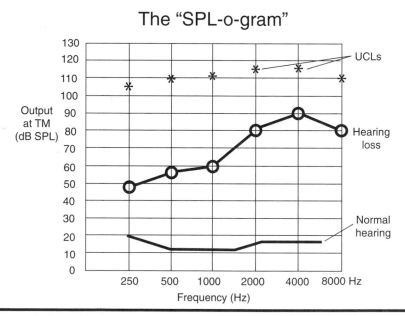

FIGURE 4–4 Unlike the typical audiogram, everything in DSL is plotted in nits of dB SPL. Normal hearing is shown as a curve, because it is now in dB SPL and the hearing loss goes up instead of down. The asterisks indicate the "ceiling" or loudness tolerance levels (LDLs) for the client. The distance between the floor (thresholds) and ceiling (LDLs) is the client's dynamic range.

along the horizontal axis and decibels along the vertical axis. Two things differ however; on the SPL-o-gram, the decibels are plotted in units of SPL, not HL. Furthermore, decibels increase upward along the vertical axis. It is worthy to note that both of these features are in keeping with the way hearing aid specifications are normally displayed. This enables everything (the hearing loss and fitting targets) to be read in the "language" of hearing aid specifications. Transferring results straight from the typical downward-going audiogram—in units of dB HL—to upward-going hearing aid hearing aid specifications—read in units of dB SPL—can (and often does) lead to a lot of confusion.

The DSL fitting method was the first to circumvent these obstacles by plotting the audiogram right-side up. At the present time, however, the NAL-NL1 fitting method has followed suit, offering a similar type of graph to display similar things. Hearing test systems, such as the Frye™ and Audioscan™ have long since evolved to incorporate the SPL-o-gram type of display.

On the SPL-o-gram, normal hearing sensitivity for one ear under a headphone is plotted in terms of dB SPL, along the bottom of the graph (Figure 4–4). The shape of the normal human audibility curve is evident, showing the typical "smile" of poorer hearing sensitivity for the low and the very high frequencies. The "floor" of right or left ear hearing loss is plotted higher up on the graph and can be readily visualized relative to normal hearing. The "ceiling" of loudness discomfort is positioned near the top of the graph as a series of asterisks. Average loudness tolerance levels as a function of frequency can be selected, or actual measured values can also be entered. It can thus be seen where the dynamic range for the client is largest and where it might become smaller. Of course, more compression will be needed for the narrow areas of the dynamic range.

There's more that sets DSL apart from its cousin fitting methods. For DSL, the *output* from the hearing aid is of final interest, not the gain. This has merit because the output, after all, is the final delivered "groceries" to the eardrum. Unlike the other fitting methods, DSL is concerned with "in situ" measures, not "insertion" measures. Insertion gain is commonly known as the difference between aided and unaided SPL at the eardrum. It does not consider or include the factors of head shadow or concha resonance, nor does it specifically address the open, unaided ear canal resonance and how it is altered when the same canal is plugged up with a piece of plastic called a "hearing aid." In situ (Latin for "in situation" or "in place") gain, on the other hand, does not exclude these factors at all because it literally surrounds them. In situ gain consists of the difference between unaided SPL at the hearing aid microphone and aided SPL at the eardrum. The DSL fitting method utilizes in situ measures because they include the factors that influence the *output* of the hearing aid on any particular person. In summary, DSL looks at output that is delivered to the eardrum, and it derives this output from the input SPL plus the in situ gain.

Unaided speech (LTASS) can also be displayed on the SPL-o-gram (Figure 4–5). Here, LTASS is superimposed across the frequencies of the hearing loss shown in Figure 4–4. It now becomes readily apparent which speech sounds sit

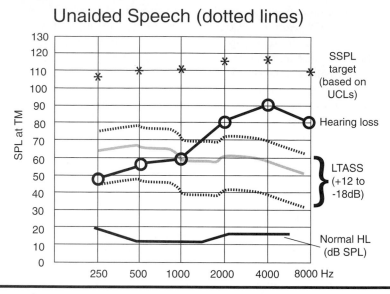

FIGURE 4-5   The long term average speech spectrum (LTASS) is plotted against the SPL-o-gram, showing the client's hearing loss and loudness tolerance levels. LTASS represents typical, unaided conversational speech intensity as a function of frequency. It generally has a 30dB dynamic range. Mean SPL is shown by the solid line; the top dotted line is 12 dB above the mean and the bottom dotted line is 18dB below the mean. Speech is thus, not a sound that is "normally" distributed around the mean. It can be seen in this example that only the low frequency portions of average spoken speech will be audible to the client; the high frequency portions will not be audible because they literally fall below the client's thresholds for those frequencies.

"below" the thresholds of the client and are thus inaudible and which speech sounds are "above" the hearing loss and are thus audible.

The goal of DSL can readily be seen on the graph: The output of the hearing aid should "raise" LTASS so that it is above the thresholds of the client and yet, so that it does not exceed the loudness tolerance levels (Figure 4-6). As we have already seen (Figure 4-3), the high-frequency elements of speech have less intensity than the more tonal, low-frequency elements do. Furthermore, most people with SNHL have poorer hearing in the high frequencies. These two factors, taken together with the stated DSL goal of making all of speech audible to the client, imply what has been stated earlier—namely, that DSL prescribes relatively more high-frequency emphasis than most other hearing aid fitting methods. As we shall see in our subsequent discussion on the NAL-NL1 fitting method, however, DSL also advocates more low-frequency output than most other fitting methods too.

The reader will notice that the mean LTASS, shown as the solid line in each figure, is not placed in the very middle of the range of LTASS, shown by the

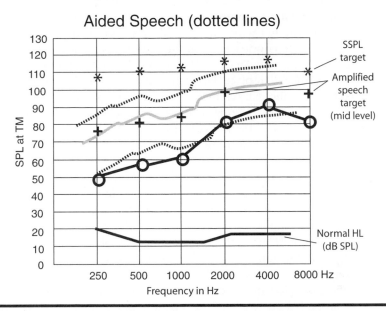

FIGURE 4–6   The DSL output target for average conversational speech (LTASS) is shown by the "+" signs. The target for amplification of average speech is situated in the client's dynamic range, between his/her thresholds and loudness tolerance levels. In other words, the goal of DSL is to literally "lift" LTASS so that it sits well within the dynamic range of the listener. Note that more compression will be required in the more narrow dynamic range at the higher frequencies.

dotted lines in each figure. This is not an accident of illustration. On the contrary, it highlights the fact that speech is a very unique sound stimulus in that its intensity fluctuates rapidly over time. Steady-state background noise, like that of a fan or air conditioner, has a fairly steady level of intensity over time. So also does the "hubbub" or "babble" of background speech in the distance. Statistically then, these types of sounds have a fairly normal distribution of intensity levels. In contrast, the intensity of close-up speech over time does not present as a normal distribution. Its mean intensity, therefore, will not necessarily fit right into the center of its range of intensity. This has implications for digital hearing aids, as will be discussed more in Chapters 7 and 8. The digital noise reduction algorithms actually capitalize or seize upon the fact that the statistical distributions of noise levels of speech are very different from those of most noises.

The DSL fitting method insists on very solid foundations of measurement to ensure the validity and reliability of the hearing aid fitting. Validity of the hearing aid fitting demands that the input is really what we think it is; only then can we have a good idea about the output from the hearing aid. A more colloquial saying from some proponents of DSL is "garbage in, garbage out." Reliability of the fitting method means that it will consistently provide the same results again and again.

The DSL fitting method attempts to account for all possible acoustic transforms that occur, beginning with the headphones used in the typical hearing test, to the standard 2cc coupler used to measure hearing aid performance, to the measurement of the actual aided SPL that is delivered to the real ear of the client with the hearing aid in place. For example, are the audiometric pure-tone test results really what the dial reading on the audiometer says they are? If the person was tested with circumaural headphones, calibrated on a 6cc coupler, then there is a lot of room for individual differences in the actual SPL that reaches the eardrum at each test frequency. The actual SPL delivered to the eardrum of the person might be very different from the dial reading on the audiometer for any test frequency. The real-ear-to-dial difference (REDD) thus has to be calculated across the frequency range. This would require real ear (probe tube) measures to be taken at each frequency, with the circum-aural headphones in place. Since almost no clinician will employ such arduous measures, DSL allows for *average* REDD values to be entered in subsequent computer target estimations. Insert headphones, on the other hand, allow less room for variability and are therefore, recommended. Furthermore, like hearing aids themselves, they are calibrated on a 2cc coupler. There is less room for acoustic transform measurement error when insert headphones are used.

The real-ear-to-coupler difference (RECD) is another factor specifically addressed in the DSL fitting method. This measure is important to consider because it affects the sound output from the hearing aid that reaches the eardrum. RECD is a measure of how the resonance of an individual real ear canal is different from that of the standard 2cc coupler used to measure hearing aid performance. The output from the receiver of the hearing aid is "sculpted" by the particular resonance of any individual's real ear canal and these changes alter the sound from the output that is given on hearing aid specification sheets. Such specifications (in North America) are derived from 2cc coupler data. It is well known, however, that predictions from hearing aid specifications do not well predict performance in an individual's actual ear. Commonly available clinical real-ear (probe tube) test equipment, such as the Frye™ and Audioscan™ enable quick RECD measurements on individual clients.

Once the client's own ear canal resonance or "ear print" is known, the RECD can be recorded and automatically factored into the equation for determining the DSL fitting targets. For the client, especially the child, this means that he or she no longer needs to be sitting in the room for subsequent probe tube (real-ear) microphone measures. The clinician can simply connect the hearing to the 2cc coupler, and factor in the client's RECD. Measures made this way allow the clinician to predict with confidence the real ear (probe tube) performance of the same hearing aid on the actual ear of the client. Additional subsequent measures (e.g., with different hearing aid trimmer settings) can also be made, and the client technically no longer needs to be present. This facet of testing could be very useful when assessing the hearing aid function on the child with a short attention span who has "better" things to do.

Instead of actually measuring the RECD, average RECD values can also be entered in the DSL computer fitting program. These values are based on norms gathered from age groups that differ by each month up to the age of 5 years. Past the age of 5 years, there is no month-to-month difference in the averaged RECD values, because the physical volume and size of the ear canal are assumed to plateau. DSL recommends actual measurement of RECD with children.

The style of hearing aid is also important to DSL, because it determines the typical resonances of the outer ear that come into play and hence, the effect of the microphone location. Microphone placements on BTE, ITE, and completely-in-canal (CIC) hearing aids are all different relative to the side of the head, the shape of the concha of the pinna, and so on. The sound input to the microphone of a hearing aid is thus, "sculpted" by its immediate surroundings. This altered input, when added to the gain of the hearing aid, will have an effect on the eventual output to the eardrum. The microphone located on the faceplate of a CIC hearing aid, for example, is buried deep inside the canal; the concha is left relatively unoccluded with a CIC than it is with a full concha shell ITE hearing aid. The sound going into the CIC microphone is, therefore, more affected by the resonance of the concha than that of the full-concha ITE. The clinician who wants to arrive at a truer estimation of hearing aid output would do well to consider the microphone location effect (MLE).

To summarize here, the three factors of REDD, RECD, and MLE form important groundwork for DSL fittings, because all of them affect the eventual output of the hearing aid at the eardrum. The DSL fitting method allows for either predicted averages or actual measured values for LDLs, REDDs, and RECDs to be entered on the fitting software. The fitting philosophy of DSL rests on these solid foundations so that the output of the hearing aid can position LTASS (unaided speech) to fit into the existing dynamic range of the client.

One last thing has yet to be discussed or shown regarding DSL: As a compression-based fitting method, it has more than one target. Common clinical implementation of DSL includes three output targets for soft, average, and loud input speech. Two case examples showing aided outputs with three different inputs are shown below.

CASE 1   **A Subject with Unusual "Cookie-Bite" Mild-to-Moderate SNHL**

This person was fit according to DSL (on the Audiocan™), with three different input SPLs: 50, 70, and 85 dB SPL (Figure 4–7). First, a sweep tone input of 70 dB SPL (at one-third octave intervals) is presented from the real-ear test equipment. This input is intended to be roughly equivalent to that of average, on-going conversational speech (LTASS). The hearing aid settings are all adjusted so that the output can best meet the target DSL output for this average speech input. Of course, it is assumed that this output is sufficient to raise LTASS above the client's thresholds. Next, a soft 40 dB SPL input level is selected. This time,

Case #1: DSL on AudioscanTM with Three Stimuli

Dotted line:	70dB SP sweep tone	average speech
Light vertical lines:	50dB SPL dynamic stimulus	soft speech
Dark vertical lines:	85dB SPL dynamic stimulus	loud speech

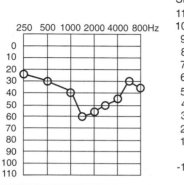

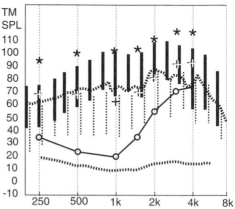

FIGURE 4–7   In this figure, the audiogram of the client is shown on the left, and the SPL-o-gram is on the right. Normal hearing is shown as the curved bottom line, the client's thresholds in dB SPL are shown as the circles, and the asterisks on top are the client's loudness tolerance levels. Aided speech, optimally amplified according to DSL targets, is placed so that most of it resides within the client's dynamic range. The DSL targets are the "+" signs, which are hidden beneath the vertical lines in this figure. Most of aided soft input speech (50dB SPL) become audible to the client, as the light vertical lines for the most part, are situated above the client's thresholds. Loud (85dB SPL) aided input speech also does not become excessively uncomfortable, because the vertical lines do not extend upwards beyond the asterisks.

however, one can choose a "dynamic" stimulus instead of a sweep tone. On the Audioscan™, the dynamic stimulus consists of a staccato-like series of bleeps of slightly different lengths and different frequencies. This is intended to imitate the stops and starts of typical speech, along with their intensity and frequency variations. Without adjusting the hearing aid output, the 50 dB dynamic input stimulus is presented. On the Audioscan™ screen, vertical lines appear, showing a range of output intensities scattered across the audiometric frequencies. Look to see if at least half of these vertical lines lie above the client's audiometric thresholds. If so, it can be assumed that at least half of soft aided speech will be audible to the client. Lastly, without adjusting the hearing aid output, present loud (85 dB SPL) dynamic input stimuli from the Audioscan™. Another set of vertical lines will appear, but these should be positioned "higher" up on the SPL-o-gram. Look to see that the tops of these vertical lines do not exceed the client's UCLs as indicated by the asterisks. This would mean that loud aided speech will not cause undue loudness discomfort for the client.

CASE 2   A Subject with a Flat SNHL

A second example of fitting soft, average, and loud speech inputs into the dynamic range of a person with a relatively flat hearing loss, with DSL, is shown in Figure 4–8. The same Audioscan™ equipment, presenting the same three inputs was used. Here, the fitting looks almost "textbook perfect," as the vertical lines fit almost completely into the dynamic range, between the "floor" (thresholds) and "ceiling" of the person's hearing loss. This would imply that almost all of soft, average, and loud aided speech sits nicely within the client's dynamic range.

Case #2: DSL on Audioscan™ with Three Stimuli

Dotted line:	70dB SP sweep tone	average speech
Lower vertical lines:	50dB SPL dynamic stimulus	soft speech
Upper vertical lines:	85dB SPL dynamic stimulus	loud speech

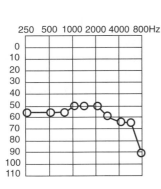
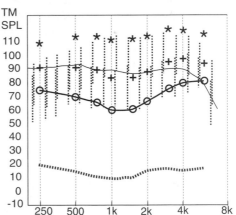

FIGURE 4–8   In this figure, soft (50dB SPL), average (70dB SPL), and loud (85 dB SPL) inputs are aided by the DSL fitting method, such that all three input levels sit neatly within the dynamic range of the client. In this fitting example, soft and loud aided speech inputs are both indicated by light vertical lines, which intersect at some frequencies. The solid line across the frequencies, above the client's thresholds, represents average aided speech inputs.

A real achievement of DSL is that audibility and comfort of aided outputs for soft, average, and loud speech inputs can be readily displayed for all to see. Contrast this to a mere insertion gain line meeting some target, as in the case of the aforementioned fitting methods covered in Chapter 3. With DSL, the projected audibility and comfort of aided speech outputs can be predicted for soft, average, and loud inputs. It is easy to see why DSL is so meaningful, especially when considering children and the acquisition of speech and language learning in the classroom. The significant implications for hearing habilitation are made obvious to the parents, teachers, and anyone else.

THE NAL-NL1 FITTING METHOD

In comparison to DSL, the NAL-NL1 fitting method is quite different. It evolved as a compression-based method in 1998, from the older NAL-R method, which is based on linear hearing aids (Chapter 3). Like all compression-based fitting methods, NAL-NL1 has more than one target, because hearing aid compression offers different gain for different input levels. Unlike the DSL fitting method, however, NAL-NL1 targets refer to gain, rather than output. As such, NAL-NL1 routinely shows three gain targets, for: 50, 65, and 80 dB SPL input levels. The gain targets for the middle inputs of 65 dB SPL are intended to represent the gain recommended for average, ongoing conversational speech inputs (Figure 4–9).

The main objective of developing NAL-NL1 was to determine the gain for several input levels that would result in maximal effective audibility (Dillon, et al., 1998a; Byrne, Dillon, Ching, Katsch, & Keidser, 2001). To calculate NAL-NL1 gain targets, gain calculations were performed for 52 people with various audiometric configurations, for input levels from 30 to 90 dB SPL, in 10 dB increments. For gently sloping, hearing loss audiograms, ranging from mild to severe in degree, the new NAL-NL1 fitting method was found to provide very similar insertion gain targets for 65 dB SPL inputs as those given by NAL-R. Consistent with the original fitting philosophy behind NAL-R (see Chapter 3), for most types of hearing loss, the mid frequencies of speech are aided so that they will sound similar in loudness to the lower and higher adjacent speech frequencies. The end aims for NAL-NL1 thus became: Equal loudness of all speech frequency bands, along with maximal speech intelligibility.

The NAL-NL1 fitting method presents with some other interesting features, which are based in part, on the original underlying philosophy of the whole NAL "family" of fitting methods (NAL, NAL-R, NAL-RP): *Equalize,* rather than preserve (or normalize), the loudness relationships among the speech frequencies. Let's examine this philosophy a bit closer. For the NAL developers, loudness "equalization" refers to amplifying adjacent speech frequency bands so that they contribute equally to the overall loudness of speech (Byrne, et al., 2001). For those with normal hearing, the low-frequency vowels are heard more loudly than the high-frequency unvoiced consonants (Figure 4–3). If this loudness relationship is preserved, then vowels will be consistently amplified so that the person with the impaired hearing who wears the hearing aids, will continue to hear the low frequency vowel sounds loudest. According to Dillon, et al. (1998b) and Bryne, et al. (2001), when other fitting methods try to preserve this normal relationship of loudness among the speech frequencies, they tend to prescribe too much gain for the low frequencies. *The NAL-NL1 fitting method does indeed prescribe less low-frequency gain than most other fitting methods. As we shall see later on, this is definitely the case with NAL-NL1 as compared to DSL.*

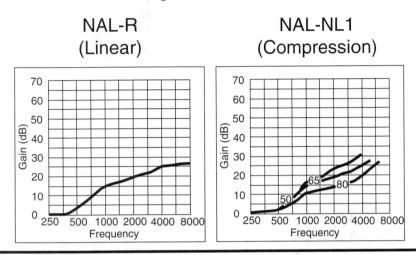

NAL-R vs NAL-NL1
Target Comparison

NAL-R
(Linear)

NAL-NL1
(Compression)

FIGURE 4–9 Note how the targets for NAL-R (left) compare to those of NAL-NL1 (right). The NAL-NL1 target for average conversational speech inputs of 65dB SPL are very similar to that of NAL-R. Even here, however, one difference appears; namely, the NAL-NL1 targets stop just beyond 4000Hz. According to NAL-NL1 fitting philosophy, aided inputs at these frequencies would not increase effective audibility.

Although normal hearing people normally hear vowels louder than high-frequency consonants, Dillon, et al. (1998b) and Byrne, et al. (2001) posit that for those with hearing loss, speech intelligibility is maximized if all of the speech frequencies of speech are equalized, rather than normalized. The only loudness that NAL strives to "normalize" (as opposed to equalize) is that of the speech spectrum as a whole; that is, all of the speech frequencies, taken together as a whole, should be amplified so that normal loudness growth is achieved. As stated by Cox (1995), sounds that are soft to the person with normal hearing should be perceived as soft to the listener with hearing aids; sounds that are comfortable for the person with normal hearing ought to be perceived as the same to the listener with hearing aids; and sounds that are loud to the person with normal hearing should be perceive as loud for the listener with hearing aids.

The reason the NAL-NL1 fitting method deviates from the approach of preserving the unaided loudness relationships among the different frequency elements of speech is because the "preserving" approach has not been shown to improve speech intelligibility (Dillon, Katsch, Byrne, Ching, Keidser, & Brewer, 1998). There is more, however, that characterizes NAL-NL1 as unique among compression-based fitting methods, and this comes from research with the older

NAL-RP intended for fitting those with severe-to-profound SNHL (Chapter 3). Recall from that discussion, that those with severe-to-profound SNHL were found to prefer more overall gain than those with lesser degrees of hearing loss (Byrne, Parkinson, & Newall, 1990). Recall also, however, that the same investigators unexpectedly discovered that those with sloping severe-to-profound hearing loss (worse hearing in the high frequencies) actually preferred *more* low-frequency gain and *less* high-frequency gain than those with the same degree of hearing loss but with a more flat hearing loss configuration. Those with the more sloping severe-to-profound SNHL thus no longer seem to want an equalized loudness across the speech frequencies. For this population, speech intelligibility was found to be maximized if the high frequencies were amplified so as to contribute less to the audible, overall loudness of speech. In other words, for this population, amplify most at frequencies where the hearing loss is the least in degree, and less where the hearing thresholds are the worst. *The implication for high-frequency targets can also then be predicted for NAL-NL1 as compared to other fitting methods; for severe high-frequency SNHL, NAL-NL1 prescribes less high-frequency gain than most other fitting methods do. Again, as we shall see later on, this is indeed the case when comparing NAL-NL1 to DSL.*

So far, we have seen that two salient features characterize the new NAL-NL1 fitting method for *compression* hearing aids: (1) the concept of equalizing, rather than normalizing the loudness of adjacent speech Hz's, and (2) providing less gain for Hz's where hearing loss is worst and more gain where hearing is best. This last point is developed further in literature describing the development of NAL-NL1, where the term "audibility" is differentiated from the term "effective audibility" (Dillon, et al., 1998a; Byrne, et al., 2001). "Audibility" can be described and measured in terms of sensation level, if actual hearing thresholds are known. "Effective audibility," on the other hand, refers to how much information can be *extracted* from speech sounds once they are audible. According to Dillon, et al. (1998a), as hearing loss increases in degree, people tend to have more "effective audibility" with less audibility. For those with severe or more hearing loss, a small sensation level might give some amount of information for understanding speech, while a greater sensation level will not necessarily add much more information. For those with profound hearing loss, audibility might be accompanied with virtually no added "effective audibility." For example, we have all encountered the client with profound HL who can hear but cannot discriminate speech without visual cues.

This finding of audibility versus effective audibility lends a salient, immediately noticeable feature to the targets of the NAL-NL1 fitting method: at times, the targets do go not completely span the audiometric frequencies (Figure 4–9). Indeed, they often end in thin air! Frequencies where the targets end are always where the hearing loss is most pronounced. For example, for reverse hearing loss figurations, NAL-NL1 targets may not appear at the very low frequencies where the hearing thresholds are greatest in degree. For sloping high-frequency hearing losses, the targets may extend from the low frequencies towards the mid frequencies, but then they may abruptly end there. According to the philosophy behind NAL-NL1, amplification at these frequencies will not contribute towards "effective audibility" with any amount of gain (Ching, 2000, personal communication; Byrne, et al. 2001).

In conclusion, although NAL-NL1 has some very different assumptions and features from those of DSL, there are several DSL features included in NAL-NL1. On their fitting software, a "speech-o-gram" includes the 30 dB dynamic range of typical, long-term unaided speech, much like DSL. In addition, the aided thresholds can be read in terms of dB SPL or HL. In keeping with the knowledge that ear canal volumes and resonances for children are far different from those of adults, the user manual for NAL-NL1 duly notes an exception in measuring insertion gain for children; here, it is suggested that RECD be measured for the purpose of reducing probe microphone measures on squirming children, but also to allow for the fact that the ear canals in children are smaller and the resonances are higher than those for adults. Last, for children, the use of real-ear-aided gain (in situ gain) is suggested instead of insertion gain, because it takes into account these unique physical characteristics when predicting what the hearing aid will actually do when on the ear of the child.

DSL versus NAL-NL1: How Do They Compare?

As we have seen, the targets for NAL-NL1 are plotted in terms of gain, while those for DSL are plotted in terms of output. To compare NAL-NL1 to DSL then, gain would have to be converted to output, or output would have to be converted to gain. For the sake of such a comparison, the author (Venema, 2002) programmed a digital hearing aid (by Unitron Hearing) on Unifit™ (the fitting software from Unitron Hearing). This software includes both the DSL and NAL-NL1 fitting methods. The Audioscan™ at the time of this comparison contained the DSL fitting method but not the NAL-NL1 fitting method. Therefore, the NAL-NL1 results had to be compared to the DSL results in terms of output. The digital hearing aid was initially programmed to best fit the output targets of DSL on Unifit™; its output was then measured and verified on the Audioscan™ real-ear probe tube test system. The same hearing aid was then programmed to best meet the gain targets of NAL-NL1 on Unifit™, and its output was then measured again on the Audioscan™. The output comparison results for DSL and NAL-NL1 on the Audioscan™ are compared here for a flat, a reverse, a sloping, and a precipitous hearing loss.

For the *flat hearing loss of 60 dB,* NAL-NL1 appears to prescribe approximately 10 dB less output than DSL, for Hz's below 1000 Hz and above 4000 Hz (Figure 4-10). The output targets for both fitting methods for the same hearing loss are very similar between 1000 and 4000 Hz. These results bear out the general expected differences, considering the philosophical differences between the two fitting methods. NAL-NL1 strives to equalize, not preserve or normalize, the loudness contributions among adjacent speech frequencies. The normally louder low-frequency vowels are amplified less with NAL-NL1, in order to make the same contribution as the amplified high-frequency consonants to the overall

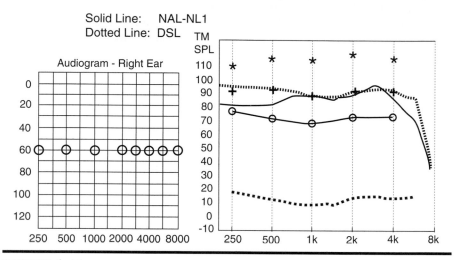

NAL-NL1 vs DSL
on Audioscan™ System

Solid Line: NAL-NL1
Dotted Line: DSL

FIGURE 4–10   The flat audiogram is shown on the left, and the output comparisons on the Audioscan™ are shown on the right. Note that the comparisons are displayed on a graph that is oriented like an "SPL-o-gram." For a flat 60dB HL audiogram, DSL prescribes some 10 dB greater output at the low frequencies than NAL-NL1, and slightly more output as well at the very high frequencies.

loudness of speech, because this would theoretically maximize the intelligibility of speech. Some slight adjustment also takes place in the high frequencies. In summary, less low-frequency and high-frequency gain is recommended by NAL-NL1.

For the reverse hearing loss, NAL-NL1 again prescribes less low-Hz output than does DSL (Figure 4–11), but this time, the difference is greater than 10 dB. Apparently, for NAL-NL1, amplification of the very worst low-frequency thresholds would not contribute much towards effective audibility. Note that NAL-NL1 actually prescribes slightly more high-Hz output than DSL for the reverse hearing loss shown here.

For the *sloping hearing loss,* NAL-NL1 and DSL appear to prescribe very similar low- and mid-Hz output (Figure 4–12). For the high frequencies, NAL-NL1 prescribes less (10–15 dB) high-Hz output than DSL. Again, for NAL-NL1, amplifying these very high frequencies, where the thresholds are the poorest, would not contribute much towards increased effective audibility.

For the *precipitous hearing loss,* NAL-NL1 and DSL appear to prescribe almost identical low- and mid-Hz output (Figure 4-13). A marked difference, however, appears for the high frequencies. NAL-NL1 prescribes a lot less high-frequency output. For severe degrees of high-frequency SNHL, the greater

NAL-NL1 vs DSL
on Audioscan™ System

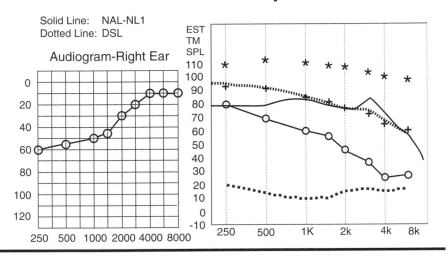

FIGURE 4–11   The reverse audiogram is shown on the left, and the output comparisons on the Audioscan™ are shown on the right. For a reverse audiogram, DSL prescribes some 10-15 dB more low frequency output than NAL-NL1.

NAL-NL1 vs DSL
on Audioscan™ System

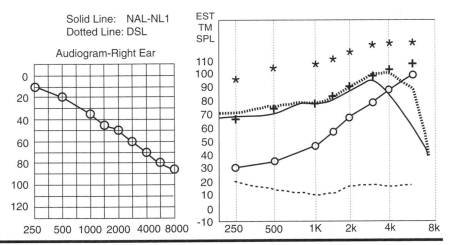

FIGURE 4–12   The sloping hearing loss is shown on the left, and the output comparisons on the Audioscan™ are shown on the right. For a sloping high frequency hearing loss audiogram, DSL prescribes 10 or more dB of high frequency output than NAL-NL1.

NAL-NL1 vs DSL
on Audioscan™ System

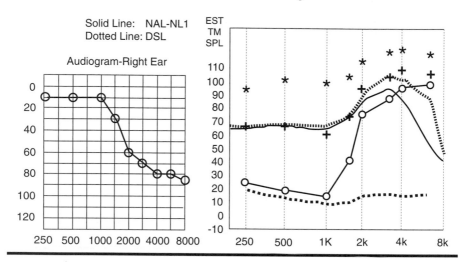

FIGURE 4–13   The sloping hearing loss is shown on the left, and the output comparisons on the Audioscan™ are shown on the right. For a precipitous, severe high frequency hearing loss, DSL again prescribes more high frequency output than NAL-NL1.

high-frequency output prescription for DSL as opposed to NAL-NL1 becomes all the more evident.

In general, for flat and for reverse hearing losses, NAL-NL1 tends to prescribe less low-Hz gain/output than DSL. For sloping and for precipitous high-frequency hearing losses, NAL-NL1 tends to prescribe less high-Hz gain/output than DSL. Based on the past record of NAL-R, the new NAL-NL1 has become an extremely popular and widely accepted fitting method for compression hearing aids. It should be appreciated that there is a psychological appeal (right, wrong, or indifferent) to being able to actually "hit" gain targets, and this is more easily accomplished with NAL-NL1 than with some other fitting methods.

Clinical reality, however, dictates that we need to face issues with facts. For example, there is a widely held, but erroneous assumption that compared to NAL-NL1, DSL is always "hungry" for high-frequency gain/output. The truth of the matter is that for most types of hearing loss the greatest difference between these two fitting methods concerns the *low* frequency gain/output. NAL-NL1 tends to prescribe less low-frequency gain than DSL. Only for the sloping to precipitous, severe, high-frequency hearing losses does DSL prescribe more high-frequency gain/output. Lastly, consider that the NAL-NL1 fitting software (Dillon, et al., 1998b) incorporates the SPL-o-gram, much as it is found on DSL fitting software (Seewald, 1997). For DSL, which originally advocated for this type of display, imitation is the finest form of flattery.

SOME REFLECTIONS ON FITTING METHODS

The plethora of hearing aid fitting formulas, as noted in Chapters 3 and 4, attests to the vastly different issue of fitting the ear versus the eye. Precious little data attest to the correctness of any one hearing aid fitting method as opposed to another. Instead, clinicians seem to be faced with the situation of learning new fitting methods as they appear or become "in vogue."

Many clinicians (the author included) were not originally trained or exposed to these kinds of fitting methods, and initially had difficulty employing them during clinical fittings. A direct comparison of required gain for most other fitting methods, as mentioned in Chapter 3 (e.g., from POGO, to NAL-R, to Berger, to Libby) is quite simple; each one of these methods offers a single target of gain that is based on some mathematical calculation or division of the audiometric thresholds. For any particular hearing loss, one can toggle between these different threshold-based methods quite easily on most real-ear test equipment, and the targets for each method can be readily visualized. On the other hand, a direct comparison between DSL and NAL-NL1 can be difficult, because DSL looks at output while NAL-NL1 defaults to look at gain. If gain is to be determined from DSL, it must be found by subtracting input levels from output levels. For those interested in simplicity, the plotting of thresholds in dB SPL, loudness tolerance levels, and the inclusion of the range of basic, unaided LTASS may also appear to clutter things somewhat.

There continues to be a huge chasm between the ideals to which some fitting methods aspire and the ideals that present "state-of-the-art" technology in hearing aids can deliver. For example, with DSL, clinicians are often dismayed by a complete inability to reach the aided output targets. Advocates often verbally point out that although this is common the main idea is to approximate the targets as closely as possible. The gulf between DSL targets and actual hearing aid responses is most often encountered when trying to fit pronounced high-frequency hearing losses.

A question that might come to mind is whether the targets, if reached, would be appreciated or accepted by the client wearing the hearing aid in the first place. Can a client always tolerate levels that would theoretically maximize their speech intelligibility? Can a fewer number of hair cells handle the acoustic load required by some of the new compression-based fitting methods? Always remember that fitting methods are a *tool* for conceptualizing a problem and solution. In keeping with this imagery, some tools are large and small wrenches, some are screwdrivers, and then there are pliers. The technology discussed in later chapters is just a means to this end. Fitting methods are a way to predict what will happen for a client with their hearing aids. But like predicting the weather, there are *many* variables to consider when predicting what hearing aids will do.

From a physiological perspective, it is not presently possible to model what is really going on in the aided cochlea with any one particular fitting method. Most clinicians fit hearing aids to the best of their abilities, but amplification at specific frequencies does not grow new hair cells. Amplification alone is not a sufficiently sophisticated tool by which to imitate the exquisite function of the cochlea. Aside from the even more coarse technology offered by cochlear implants, however, amplification is all that is available. Aided sound outputs are driven through a middle ear system with the intention of increasing the traveling wave amplitude and the stimulation of damaged and missing hair cells. The technology of WDRC is meant to imitate the role of the outer hair cells, which are thought to help the inner hair cells sense soft sounds. Hearing aids, however, cannot presently *sharpen* the traveling wave, as the outer hair cells are thought to do. Although our hearts might be in the right place, we are still "picking up needles with mittens on."

The art and the science of clinical hearing aid fittings are complementary facets. In particular, it can be very difficult for clinicians to make the transition from linear-based to compression-based fitting methods, and to decide which fitting method to use. Furthermore, there is a large chasm between the ideals of some hearing aid fitting methods and the deliverable realities of most hearing aid circuits. With these situations, the clinical fitting of hearing aids remains both an art and a science.

Hearing aids, even the most sophisticated digital hearing aids, are a coarse, gross approximation of an exquisitely fine-tuned cochlea. This is why the term hearing "aid" is not such a bad one. A hearing aid for an ear is like a cane for a bad knee; it helps, but it cannot replace the real thing. We can no more restore normal cochlear function with a hearing aid than we can replace an amputated hand with an artificial one.

Fitting methods should not be put ahead of a client's needs, nor should they be held up as banners of one's stance in a holy war against peers who may use different methods. As discussed in Chapter 3, the whole field of clinical hearing aid fitting is not as purely scientific as we sometimes want to think it is. It may be a good idea to consider the targets of fitting methods, as goals to eventually achieve. A new elderly client may not initially accept the amount of gain or output suggested by DSL; in such a case, it may be a good idea to start off by fitting this client with a method that asks for less gain (e.g., NAL-NL1). On the other hand, an infant has not yet acquired speech and language. Should we not then ensure to the best of our abilities, that soft, high-frequency unvoiced consonants become audible here? The fitting method used should depend on what the goals are. Perhaps clinicians should not slavishly adhere to any one particular fitting method for all cases.

For Mrs. McGillicudy who has presbycusis, however, what is the upshot of fitting a hearing aid with one method versus another? What really constitutes a good hearing aid fitting? Are we really doing what we say we are doing when we fit hearing aids with one method versus another? Unlike optometry, various hearing aid fitting strategies abound in our field, but the benefits of each fitting method are not clearly defined. People do not develop a splitting headache or stand a greater chance of driving a car into a tree when fit with NAL-R versus DSL. Hearing aids and people still mix like oil and water. Issues like sound quality and speech intelligibility come into the picture, but it is the clinician's skill at both the art and science of fitting hearing aids that still remains at the heart of the matter.

SUMMARY

- Loudness growth, compression circuitry in hearing aids, and compression-based fitting methods all fit together.

- The thresholds of SNHL are worse than those of normal hearing, yet loudness tolerance is usually not much different from that of normal hearing. Instead of thinking of hearing loss thresholds as a below normal plot on an audiogram, it may help to flip the audiogram upside-down, and think of them as the "floor" of hearing sensitivity being raised compared to that of normal hearing. Similarly, loudness tolerance can be seen as the "ceiling." In this way, we can consider the dynamic range being smaller than normal for hearing loss. A smaller dynamic range means a faster growth of loudness.

- Compression circuitry, unlike linear circuitry, changes the gain depending on the input intensity level. Compression, in general, gives a greater gain for soft input intensity levels, and less gain for more intense inputs. Soft input sounds below the "floor" of the hearing thresholds need to be amplified by a lot, while intense sounds that are near the "ceiling" do not need to be amplified by much at all. For those with smaller-than-normal dynamic ranges and consequently, faster-than-normal loudness growths, compression hearing aids may provide a better fit than linear hearing aids.

- Compression-based fitting methods are based on restoring normal loudness growth with compression hearing aids. They all focus on speech as the target, which has its own unique properties, and they try to fit amplified speech into the smaller-than-normal dynamic range of the person with hearing loss.

- The DSL and NAL-NL1 fitting methods were compared in this chapter. The DSL fitting method, developed in Canada at the University of Western Ontario, originated the SPL-o-gram, plots output (not gain) targets, and its focus is on the audibility and comfort of aided speech. The NAL-NL1 fitting method, developed in Australia, at the National Acoustics Laboratories, equalizes (not normalizes) the loudness of speech, meaning that it tries to make all speech frequency bands contribute equally towards the overall loudness (audibility) of speech. As such, it prescribes relatively less low-frequency gain/output than DSL. It also addresses the concept of "effective audibility" or the meaning that one can derive from audible speech. For severe high-frequency SNHL, very little effective audibility can be derived from the severely damaged hair cells representing the high frequencies. For these hearing losses, therefore, NAL-NL1 prescribes less high-frequency gain/output than DSL.

REVIEW QUESTIONS

1. A normal dynamic range is closest to:
   a. 50 dB.
   b. 75 dB.
   c. 100 dB.
   d. 125 dB.

2. Fitting methods that assume linear gain tend to provide _____ target(s).
   a. one
   b. two
   c. three
   d. four

3. A reduced dynamic range most often means worse hearing thresholds and:
   a. greater-than-normal loudness tolerance.
   b. reduced loudness tolerance.
   c. similar-to-normal loudness tolerance.
   d. very poor speech discrimination.

4. The DSL fitting methods plots its targets in terms of:
   a. input.
   b. gain.
   c. output.
   d. none of the above

5. The DSL fitting method originates from _____; the NAL-NL1 fitting method originates from:
   a. USA / Lithuania
   b. Canada / USA
   c. Australia / USA
   d. Canada / Australia

6. To restore normal loudness growth for moderate SNHL, a hearing aid should amplify:
   a. soft sounds by a lot, and loud sounds by little or nothing at all.
   b. loud sounds by a lot, and soft sounds by little or nothing at all.
   c. all input sounds by exactly the same amount.
   d. none of the above

7. What is missing from the loudness growth model shown in Figure 4–1?
   a. intensity
   b. psycho-acoustic perceptions
   c. frequency
   d. dynamic range

8. The focus of DSL is:
   a. high-frequency gain.
   b. equalized loudness for all speech frequencies.
   c. effective audibility of speech.
   d. audibility of speech.

9. In situ gain is the difference between:
   a. aided and unaided SPL at the eardrum.
   b. unaided sound at the hearing aid microphone and aided SPL at the eardrum.
   c. aided and unaided thresholds.
   d. none of the above

10. For a flat, moderate SNHL, NAL-NL1 prescribes ____ and ____ than DSL.
   a. less low- and less high-frequency gain
   b. more low- and more high-frequency gain
   c. less low- and more high-frequency gain
   d. more low- and less high-frequency gain

RECOMMENDED READINGS

Florentine, M. (2003). It's not recruitment – gasp! It's softness imperception. *The Hearing Journal, 56*(3), 10–15.

Mueller, G. H. (1997). 20 questions: Prescriptive fitting methods: The next generation. *The Hearing Journal, 50*(10), 10–19.

  This reference cites several other sources. It also gives the phone numbers, faxes, and Internet addresses for ordering any of the fitting methods described in this chapter.

REFERENCES

Byrne, D., Dillon, H., Ching, T., Katsch, R., and Keidser, G. (2001). NAL-NL1 procedure for fitting nonlinear hearing aids: Characteristics and comparisons with other fitting methods. *Journal of the American Academy of Audiology, 12,* 37–51.

Byrne, D., Parkinson,A., and Newall, P. (1990). Hearing aid gain and frequency response requirements for the severely/profoundly hearing impaired. *Ear and Hearing, 11,* 40–49.

Cornelisse, L. E., Gagne, J. P., & Seewald, R. C. (1991). Ear-level recordings of the long-term average spectrum of speech. *Ear and Hearing, 12,* 47–54.

Cornelisse, L. E., Seewald, R. C., & Jamieson, D. G. (1994). Wide-dynamic-range compression hearing aids: The DSL[i/o] approach. *The Hearing Journal, 47*(10): 23–29.

Cox, R. M. (1995). Using loudness data for hearing aid selection: The IHAFF approach. *The Hearing Journal, 48*(2): 10–44.

Cox, R. M., and Moore, J. N. (1988). Composite speech spectrum for hearing aid gain prescriptions. *Journal of Speech and Hearing Research,* 31, 102–107.

Dillon, H., Katsch, R., Byrne, D., Ching, T., Keidser, G., & Brewer, S. (1998a). The NAL-NL1 prescription procedure for non-linear hearing aids. *National Acoustics Laboratories Research and Development, Annual Report* 1997/98, pp 4–7.

Dillon, H., Byrne, D., Brewer, S., Katsch,, R., Ching, T., and Keidser, G. (1998b). *NAL Nonlinear Version 1.01 User Manual.* Chatswood, Australia: National Acoustics Laboratories.

Florentine, M. (2003). It's not recruitment—gasp! It's softness imperception. *The Hearing Journal,* 56(3): 10–15.

Killion, M. C. (1997). The SIN report: Circuits haven't solved the hearing-in-noise problem. *The Hearing Journal, 50*(10): 28–34.

Seewald, R. (1992). The desired sensation level method for fitting children: Version 3.0. *The Hearing Journal, 45*(5): 36–41.

Seewald, R. C. (1997). Amplification: A child-centered approach. *The Hearing Journal, 50*(3): 61.

Venema, T. (2002). The NAL-NL1 fitting method. *The Hearing Professional,* July–August

Yost, W. A. (2000). *Fundamentals of hearing: An introduction* (4th ed.). San Diego: Academic Press, Inc.

5

The Many Faces of Compression

INTRODUCTION

Compression is the big word today in the realm of hearing aids. At almost every conference that has to do with hearing, there is some presentation that deals specifically with the issues of compression. Towards the end of the decade of the 1990s, hearing aid specifications all hailed the advent and eminence of compression, and all kinds of compression hearing aids began to be sold by almost every hearing aid manufacturer. Here at this point, it must be emphasized that the decade of the 1990s witnessed the flourishing of compression advances at the tail end of the reign of analog hearing aids. At the present time, almost all hearing aids sold are digital. These, too, utilize the same types of compression; however, they do so with digital software algorithms instead of the exclusive use of resistors, capacitors, and other physical electrical components.

Today, most digital hearing aids are adjusted (or digitally programmed) by means of the fitting software provided by their specific manufacturers. Many clinicians choose a general "quick-fit" option to adjust a digital hearing aid to best fit a client's particular hearing loss configuration. When clinicians select this kind of fitting option, however, the compression characteristics of the digital hearing aid are sometimes buried under the surface, nowhere to be seen on the screen. The specific compression characteristics of the digital hearing aids are more often seen when a more specific fitting option is selected. It should be noted that in many instances, even the paper hearing aid specification sheets, published by the hearing aid manufacturers, sometimes omit many of the compression specifics of today's digital hearing aids.

It is as if the decade of the 1990s was the "golden" age of compression. Almost all hearing aids were analog hearing aids, and these were comprised of one specific type of compression or another. Wide dynamic range compression (WDRC) was beginning to emerge, seasoned clinicians were put into the position of having to learn it as a new type of compression, and manufacturers regularly held seminars where compression types were outlined, explained, and compared.

At that time, clinicians could often adjust the compression by the trimmer of the hearing aid; however, changing to another *type* of compression meant choosing another hearing aid. Today's digital hearing aids still include the same types of compression, but we now have the ability to almost completely select the compression type(s) and also sculpt the compression characteristics themselves with the fitting software. The ease of programming today's digital hearing aids by means of programming software has thus actually served to cloud clinicians' understanding of compression itself.

To understand why and how certain types of compression are employed for different degrees of hearing loss and for various clinical fitting populations, we must understand the various types of compression. Anything less makes the clinician a blind follower of manufacturer fitting software. To appreciate compression types as they are combined in today's digital hearing aids, it behooves the clinician to understand compression types as they once stood alone in yesterday's analog hearing aids. This chapter sets out to explain and describe each type of compression separately, as they used to be offered in yesterday's analog hearing aids. It is hoped that this chapter will help clinicians understand the rationale behind the same types of compression found in today's digital hearing aids.

In the 1990s, many graduate programs in audiology were guilty of not teaching compression very well, often because the professor of the one hearing aids class offered in those programs did not really understand compression. Those were the days when the manufacturers had most of this kind of knowledge, and the universities were generally "out of it." Those days have changed; most Audiology and Hearing Instrument Specialist programs offer at least two hearing aids classes, where compression is covered quite well. Over time, however, this knowledge can become dull. Many clinicians using the "quick fit" options on the fitting software may lose their sound grasp on the many types of compression, and when to fit what type.

In the preceding chapters the cochlea was presented as a magnificent nonlinear organ. Our attempts to restore "normal" hearing with imperfect technology and a myriad of fitting methods have met with limited success. Although we are taking small steps toward our goal, they *are* in the right direction. This chapter explains the technical areas of compression in hearing aids. In Chapter 6, we will look at multi-channel and programmability. In Chapter 7, we will discuss how these elements of compression are combined together in today's digital hearing aids. In Chapter 8, we will examine the features of directional microphones and digital noise reduction, and compare the clinical benefits of each.

Compression has many faces. There is no one simple way to describe it cleanly. The best way to look at compression is like we do when we look at a sculpture. One needs to walk around it and see it from several different angles to appreciate it. This chapter aims at doing just that.

At the outset, it should be mentioned that there are essentially three real building blocks of compression, much like the X, Y, and Z dimensions of compression; these are the separate but inter-related concepts of: 1. input versus output compression, 2. the effects of different trimmers for adjusting compression, and 3. compression that focuses on limiting the ceiling (output limiting compression) versus compression that focuses on lifting the floor (WDRC). Bass and treble increases at low levels. BILL and TILL are two "children" of WDRC, and many multi-channel, programmable hearing aids utilize both of these aspects. Dynamic aspects of compression consist of the attack/release times that can be encountered (and selected, for that matter) in today's compression hearing aids. These are the specific areas to be covered in this chapter.

A WORD ABOUT INPUT/OUTPUT GRAPHS

Input/output graphs are the most common way to explain compression, and they can appear on any specs sheet from any hearing aid manufacturer, so it may be a good idea to make them your friends. Ideally, clinicians should be able to ignore the written content on the specs sheets from any hearing aid manufacturer, look only at the graphs, and be able to tell what type of compression is being shown.

The graphs in many of the following figures are input/output graphs, with the X axes showing input sound pressure level (SPLs) and the Y axes showing output SPLs. The diagonal lines on each graph are the "functions" and they represent the working of the hearing aid. The functions on each graph show the *difference* between corresponding input and output levels; in other words, the functions show the *gain* of a hearing aid for different input SPLs.

Notice that on input/output graphs, the values of input and output are always expressed as "dB SPL." This is because they are each referenced to some absolute value, representing 0 dB SPL (e.g., this could be 0.0002 dynes/cm2). Whenever gain is the value of interest, the reader might notice it expressed simply as "dB." This is because gain is a *relative* decibel value that is not referenced to any specific sound pressure representing 0 dB SPL. The reader might recall being specifically taught that one cannot simply arithmetically add decibel values together; this is true for adding two decibel values that are each separately referenced to some *absolute* pressure representing 0 dB SPL. One *can* simply add dB values together (or subtract dB from one another, for that matter) if simply adding a *relative* dB value to an absolute dB value that is referenced to .0002 dynes/cm2. For example, a 30 dB conductive hearing loss + 30 dB SNHL = 60 dB total mixed hearing loss. For another example, an input of 50 dB SPL plus a gain of 50 dB equals a total output of 100 dB SPL. This is an often overlooked fact when discovering the decibel. In our field, we often *do indeed* simply add decibel values together!

As discussed in Chapter 3, the most important formula for understanding hearing aid function is: input + gain = output. For most input/output graphs, linear gain is represented by the 45° diagonal lines. The point where each gain line suddenly takes a bend is called the compression "threshold," or "kneepoint," and it is at this point that "compression" begins. The "kneepoint" of compression above the input axis shows the input SPL where compression begins. From now on, the term "kneepoint" is used to describe the input where compression begins.

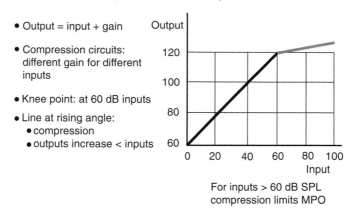

Compression Amplification

- Output = input + gain

- Compression circuits: different gain for different inputs

- Knee point: at 60 dB inputs

- Line at rising angle:
  - compression
  - outputs increase < inputs

For inputs > 60 dB SPL compression limits MPO

FIGURE 5–1   With compression hearing aids, the output increases in a linear fashion, entirely along with the input, up until the kneepoint. The kneepoint is the bend in the line function on the input/output graph. Beyond (to the right of) the kneepoint, the output still increases with input increases, but this increase is no longer at a corresponding 1:1 rate. It is at this point, that compression begins. In this example, the compression ratio is 4:1, which means that 4 dB input increases are accompanied with only 1 dB output increases. Contrast this situation to that of linear peak clipping, as shown in Figure 3-3. With peak clipping, the output increases stop abruptly. That is, further input increases do not result in any further output increases. In this example, the gain of the compression hearing aid is 60 dB. For 20 dB inputs, the output is 80 dB; for 60 dB inputs, the output is 120 dB; this is still linear gain. For 80 dB inputs, however, the output is 125 dB, because with a 4:1 compression ratio, a 20 dB input increase results in a 5 dB output increase. Similarly, for a 100 dB input, the output is 130 dB SPL.

The gain shown in many input/output graphs is linear to the left of (or below) the kneepoint, which means that for any increase of input SPL there is a correspondingly equal increase of output SPL. For example, if the hearing aid has a gain of 60 dB, then a 10 dB SPL input will result in a 70 dB SPL output, a 20 dB SPL input results in an 80 dB SPL output, and so on (Figure 5-1). Linear gain was discussed in Chapter 3.

Contrast now, compression shown in Figure 5-1 to linear gain, shown in Figure 3-3, Chapter 3. The linear hearing aid example in Figure 3-3 has a gain of 60 dB and a maximum power output (MPO) of 120 dB SPL. Note in that example, that at an input level of 60 dB SPL, the output suddenly no longer increased along with the input. For input levels greater than 60 dB SPL, the linear hearing aid went into "peak clipping," and the maximum power output (MPO) remained at 120 dB SPL. Now take a look at Figure 5-1, which shows compression instead of linear gain. For the sake of consistency, the gain in this example is still 60 dB; furthermore, at input levels beyond 60 dB SPL, something again happens. This time, however, it is not peak clipping but rather, *compression* that occurs. Note how the MPO does not take a straight horizontal direction to the right; instead, it rises at a more shallow slope. In this example, the MPO is limited with a bit of "give." Instead of hitting one's head against a cement ceiling, it's as if some sponge was attached to the cement ceiling, thus softening the thud. In fact, that is how the first compression came to be; it was a method of limiting the MPO without the distortion caused by peak clipping! More will be discussed on output limiting later on in this chapter, under the heading "Output Limiting."

With compression, the gain is "nonlinear" because the gain *changes* as a function of input SPL. The hearing aid provides linear gain (where the gain function is at a 45° angle) until input levels seen below the kneepoint are reached; above that intensity level, compression begins. When there is compression, an increase in input SPL does *not* correspond to an equal increase in the output SPL. On the contrary, the gain for input SPLs "above" or to the right of the kneepoint is *less* than the gain for input SPLs "below" the kneepoint. The slope of any line to the right of a compression kneepoint shows the effect of compression on the gain of the hearing aid (Figure 5–1). A compression kneepoint, for example, at an input of 60 dB SPL means that the hearing aid provides linear gain for input levels up to 60 dB SPL. For inputs above that intensity level, compression begins. In most cases, compression is visualized on input-output graphs as a diagonal line that is more shallow in slope or slant that the 45° angle line where linear gain is seen. The more shallow the slope, the greater the amount of compression.

For input sound pressure levels to the right of or above the kneepoint, compression thus, determines the MPO of the hearing aid. The MPO is shown by the general "height" of any line that is to the right of the kneepoint. Always remember that compression is really a gain-related issue. Only with regard to input, does compression affect the sum total MPO. Thus, on input/output graphs showing compression, for input sound pressure levels to the right of (or above) the kneepoint, compression determines the MPO of the hearing aid.

Compression ratios are the *amount* of compression provided by the hearing aid once compression begins. Compression ratios can be visualized on an input/output graph by the slant of the line after the kneepoint. A 10:1 compression ratio means that for every 10 dB increase of input SPL, there is only a 1 dB corresponding increase to the output SPL. A 2:1 compression ratio means that for every 10 dB increase of input SPL, there is a corresponding 5 dB increase to the output SPL of the hearing aid. Higher compression ratios indicate *more* compression, that is, progressively *less* gain than linear gain.

In summary, for the subsequent input/output graphs you will encounter, it is helpful to see the 45° angle lines as representing linear gain; the shallower lines that continue on to the right of the kneepoint can be seen as representing the MPO as controlled by compression. Think of the kneepoint as the "when" of compression, and the ratio as the "how much" of compression. Compression is often referred to as automatic gain control (AGC), because the gain of the hearing aid changes as the input intensity SPL changes.

Some hearing aids provide what is known as "curvilinear compression." This refers to the corner of the input/output line or function (Figure 5–2). Instead of

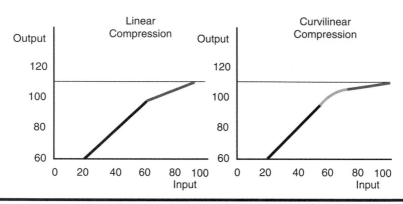

Curvilinear Compression

FIGURE 5–2   "Linear" compression is shown on the left and curvilinear compression is shown on the right. Although the terms might be confusing, it might be helpful to note that for linear compression, the kneepoint is sharply defined and the compression taking place to the right of the kneepoint is a linear function (a straight line). This results in a constant compression ratio. For curvilinear compression, the kneepoint is rounded and less defined, and the compression ratio actually changes with changes inputs.

having a sharp bend, the line takes a curve. The kneepoint is rounded instead of having a sharp corner. Curvilinear compression shows that the hearing aid *gradually* goes into its full degree or amount of compression; that is, the amount of compression increases gradually over increasing input levels.

INPUT COMPRESSION VERSUS OUTPUT COMPRESSION

When the clinician is confronted with compression, the first division that becomes apparent is the issue of input compression versus output compression. What is the difference and, furthermore, when does one fit which type? Input versus output compression can be considered the "X" dimension of compression. When I once taught compression late in hearing aids class at a university some 10 years ago, I said that input compression hearing aids have a compressor located between the microphone and the amplifier and that output compression hearing aids have a compressor located between the amplifier and the receiver. Whether this is true or not is one thing; but it is of precious little value to the clinician fitting Mrs. McGillicudy who has presbycusis.

For the clinician, the big difference between input and output compression is where the where the *volume control* (VC) is in the circuit (see bottom of Figure 5-3), and what it consequently *does* (see top of Figure 5-3) because *it* is manipulated by the person who wears the hearing aid (at least on traditional

Imput versus Output Compression: Volume Control Effects

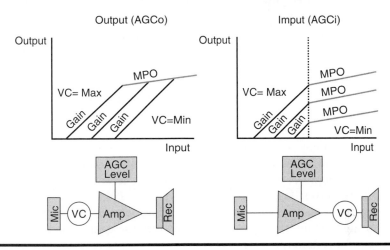

FIGURE 5–3 Input/output graphs and simple circuit schematics showing relative volume control positions for output compression (left) and input compression (right). For each graph, the parallel diagonal lines rising from the X axis represent linear gain; the corners represent the threshold kneepoint of compression; the line(s) to the right of the kneepoints represent the maximum power output (MPO). The position of the volume control in the circuits determines its effect. For output compression (left), the volume control affects gain and kneepoint, but not MPO. For input compression (right), the volume control affects gain and MPO, but not kneepoint.

hearing aid styles having user-controlled VCs; some hearing aids don't even have VCs). If the VC has a different effect for input than it does for output compression, it behooves of the clinician to know what that difference is.

For analog output compression hearing aids, the VC was literally situated "early on" in the circuit; it was located between the microphone and the amplifier (Figure 5-3, bottom left). For input compression hearing aids, the VC was situated almost dead last in the circuit, just in front of the receiver that sends sound into the ear (Figure 5-3, bottom right).

Different VC locations lead to dramatic differences in what they do. The two graphs in Figure 5-3 show the different effects of the VCs with output compression hearing aids (top left) and input compression hearing aids (top right).

In today's digital hearing aids, digital algorithms can mathematically imitate or mimic the effects of different physical VC locations in analog circuits. In this way, a digital hearing aid does not have to be locked into being either input or output compression. The programming software of the digital hearing aid can simply create the effects of input or output compression.

Output Compression

For output compression hearing aids (Figure 5–3, top left), the VC affects the gain but not the MPO. The three 45° diagonal gain lines in each graph show the effects of three different VC positions upon the gain of the hearing aid. The right-most line actually shows minimum gain, with the volume control position *lowered* to a minimum position. The left-most line shows maximum gain, with the volume control *raised* to a maximum position.

To make this clear, it may help to draw some more lines here. From the right-most kneepoint on the output compression graph, draw a vertical line down to the input axis. From the same kneepoint, draw a horizontal line to the output axis. This shows that at the minimum volume control setting, some X amount of input is needed to give some Y amount of output. If similar vertical and horizontal lines are drawn from the left-most kneepoint, it may become clear that for the maximum volume control position, less input is needed to give about the same amount of output. At low-volume positions, lots of input is needed to result in some amount of output. At high-volume positions, less input is needed to give about the same amount of output. This means that the gain is increased as the volume control position is raised.

The input/output graph also shows that once "past" or to the right of the kneepoint, in the region of compression, there is only one MPO line that is common to all three diagonal lines. This shows that, for output compression hearing aids, the volume control does not affect the MPO. Output compression is thus very suitable for *high-power* hearing aids, because for these hearing aids, clinicians should be very concerned about providing excessive output that can potentially damage hearing even further.

Note that the VC also changes the compression kneepoint. In analog hearing aids this is because the compression kneepoint is adjusted "later on" in the circuit after the volume control; the compressor is always set to wait for some steady amount of voltage that will tell it to compress (Figure 5–3, bottom left). The volume control affects the amount of input signal that will arrive at the compressor of the hearing aid. If this amount of input voltage is not enough to tell the compressor to compress, then it will not act. Only when the VC sends the required input signal voltage that the compressor is "waiting for," will the compressor then "do its thing." Again, in today's digital hearing aids, these action are mimicked mathematically in the digital software algorithms.

Input Compression

For input compression hearing aids the effects of the VC are completely different (see Figure 5–3, top right). For input compression, the volume control affects both the gain *and* the MPO. Again, three diagonal gain lines for three different volume control positions are shown. Once again, the right-most 45° diagonal gain line shows the lowest volume control setting, and the left-most gain line shows the highest or maximum volume control setting. It is obvious that the

Input versus Output Compression: Volume Control Effects on Frequency Response

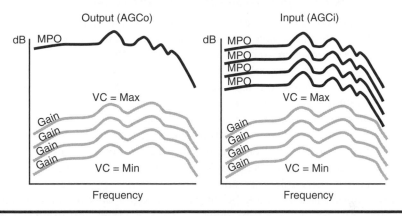

FIGURE 5–4 Frequency responses showing relative volume control positions for output compression (left) and input compression (right). Again, as shown in Figure 4-1, the volume control for output compression adjusts the gain, but not the MPO; for input compression, the volume control adjusts the gain along with the MPO.

MPO is also affected by the volume control because once "past" or to the right of the kneepoint, the height of all three gain lines also changes.

There is no specific, intended design feature or clinical fitting advantage to have the VC affect the MPO on input compression hearing aids. Rather, on analog hearing aids, this feature was simply a by-product of the VC placement in the circuit. In addition, the VC placed early on in the circuit simply allowed for another control—the TK control—to be placed near the end of the circuit (more on this control will be described later on in the next section). At any rate, those with mild-to-moderate SNHL have a larger dynamic range than those with severe SNHL and can more easily accommodate an MPO that rides up and down with VC adjustments. Input compression hearing aids are therefore, often moderate-power hearing aids, intended for mild-moderate SNHL

Note also for input compression hearing aids, that the VC does not affect the kneepoint of compression. As Figure 5-3 (bottom right) shows, the compressor is situated before the VC. This means that the VC does nothing to the kneepoint because the compression kneepoint is already determined!

Input/output graphs are not the only way to look at the differences in the VC effects. The clinician is apt to be familiar with the frequency responses (gain as a function of frequency) seen on a hearing aid test box screen or printout, as shown in Figure 5-4. Here, the effects of the VC on gain and MPO are readily apparent for output compression (left graph) in comparison to input compression (right graph). For output compression, the VC increases and decreases the gain; for input compression, both the gain and the MPO are affected by the VC.

Clinical Uses of Input and Output Compression

Input and output compressions are not "better" or "worse" than each other; they are just different, and they have different clinical applications. Output compression may be good for severe-to-profound SNHL where the dynamic range is very small. For these clients, the clinician may worry that an excessively high VC position might cause damage to remaining hair cells or residual hearing; an output compression circuit will ensure that the VC affects only the gain and not the MPO. For the same reason, on older analog hearing aids, which were either output or input compression, output compression was also often selected for use on children. The parent, teacher, or caregiver did not need to worry about excessive MPO causing further hearing loss, when the little person ran into the house with the VC on a full-on position.

Input compression in analog hearing aids was generally recommended for mild-to-moderate SNHL where the dynamic range is larger and there is consequently more room for "play" on MPO. Again, input compression in analog hearing aids also allowed for the use of the TK compression control, which was of special use for those with mild to moderate SNHL. As we have seen in Chapter 1, mild-to-moderate presbycusis is the most common type of hearing loss. Input compression hearing aids thus had a large potential fitting application. *Today, most digital hearing aids incorporate the use of input compression for soft inputs, along with output compression for louder inputs.*

In addition to testing each type of compression on a hearing aid test box, one can also *hear* the effects of output versus input compression (the cochlea is an excellent acoustic analyzer). To hear the differences between output and input compression, talk softly into each hearing aid while adjusting the VC; with both output and input compression one should notice the volume go up and down, because the VC adjusts the gain on both. Now talk loudly into each while adjusting the VC; the volume should change mostly when listening to the input compression hearing aid, because only on these hearing aids does the VC adjust the MPO.

COMPRESSION CONTROLS: CONVENTIONAL VERSUS "TK"

The issue of input and output compression can be left in the "rear view mirror" and we can turn now to another face of compression, the effect of manipulating another variable in hearing aids—namely, the compression kneepoint control. For this topic or "Y" dimension of compression, think of the variable of VC as frozen in a constant position.

There are two types of compression kneepoint controls: (1) the earliest or original type, here called the output limiting compression control, and (2) a compression control originally developed for hearing aids in the late 1980s,

Different Ways of Adjusting Compression

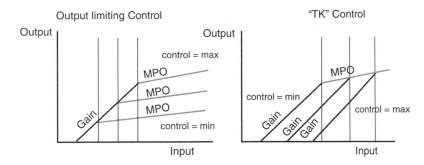

Output limiting control: Affects Kneepoint & Output
"TK" control: Affects Kneepoint & Gain

FIGURE 5–5 Input/output graphs showing effects of two different types of compression controls (volume control is assumed to be held constant at some position). For both graphs, the diagonal line(s) rising from the X axis represent the linear gain; the corners represent the threshold kneepoint of compression; the line(s) to the right of the kneepoints represent the maximum power output (MPO). Both controls adjust the kneepoint of compression, but that is where the similarity ends. The conventional compression control affects MPO, although the TK control affects gain for soft input sound pressure levels only.

commonly known as the threshold kneepoint (TK) control. The effect of each of these can be seen in Figure 5-5. Both graphs in the figure are once again, input/output graphs, similar to those in Figure 5-3.

Conventional Compression Control

The left graph in Figure 5-5 shows the effects of the output limiting compression kneepoint control. It is typically found in conjunction with output compression. When hearing aids were all analog, there were *some* input compression hearing aids that also utilized the output limiting compression control. Again, it should be appreciated that in the decade of the 1980s, when compression first appeared in hearing aids, this type of control was used as a way to limit the MPO without the distortion caused by peak clipping. Therefore, all hearing aids with compression—either output or input—utilized this type of compression control. Toward the middle of the 1990s, the analog *input* compression hearing aids began to utilize a different kind of compression control—the "TK" control. More will be discussed on this control later in this section. For now, let's look at the specific function of the output limiting type of compression control.

The output limiting compression control affects the compression kneepoint and the MPO. It does so by adjusting the voltage level that the compressor of the circuit needs to begin compressing. As the control is turned to a maximum position, the compression kneepoint is raised, along with the MPO. At a maximum kneepoint setting, the compression hearing aid is actually in a linear (1:1) gain mode for a wide range of soft to average input SPLs; compression will not occur until input sounds that are higher than the intensity level specified by the kneepoint are reached. At this maximum kneepoint setting, the MPO is also increased. Note from Figure 5–5 (left-most graph) that the conventional compression control does *not* affect the gain; because the 45° diagonal, linear gain line does *not* change in position with changes to the compression control settings.

The effects of this control can be heard in addition to being tested on a hearing aid test box (the cochlea is an excellent acoustic analyzer). To hear the effect of this compression control, you must speak *loudly* into the hearing aid, because only then will the input sound plus the gain reach the MPO (a low-intensity input sound, such as a soft voice, plus the gain of the hearing aid may not result in an output that reaches the MPO). As the compression control is turned from a maximum position to a minimum position, the kneepoint of compression as well as the MPO are reduced; one should notice that the amplified loud voice becomes softer. This is because the compression control affects the MPO, not the gain.

TK Control

The TK control is completely different. On analog hearing aids, it emerged as a type of compression control much later than the original output limiting type of compression control. Many clinicians during the 1990s were initially confused by the TK control because it works so very differently from the output limiting compression control. On digital hearing aids today, the TK control works the same way, but it may not always be called a "TK" control. It may be seen on digital software as adjusting the left-most, or lower, kneepoint on a rather complex looking input/output graph. More will be specifically described about compression in digital hearing aids per se, in the next chapter (7). For now, let's simply look at the TK control and how it works in general.

The right-most graph in Figure 5–5 shows the effect of the TK control. Technically, any compression control affects the kneepoint of compression, but electrical engineers will probably be quick to note that the term "threshold kneepoint" is an input-related term, and rarely encountered with output compression hearing aid circuitry. At any rate, the TK control is always found in conjunction with input compression, more specifically, with a certain subset of input compression known as "wide dynamic range compression" (WDRC), which we will discuss in the next section. In older analog hearing aids, the TK control was first associated with hearing aids using the KAmp™ circuit. Along with that circuit, the TK control began to be known as a separate entity from the conventional output limiting type of compression control.

The TK control affects the threshold kneepoint of compression and also the gain for *soft* input SPLs below 60 dB SPL. This is because the TK control adjusts the kneepoint of compression over a range of relatively low input levels, from around 40 to 60 dB SPL. Like all compression hearing aids, those with the TK control provide greater linear gain below the threshold kneepoint of compression. However, because this kneepoint is found at relatively soft inputs, the TK control can be seen as a gain booster for soft sounds. Unlike the conventional compression control, the TK control does not affect the MPO.

The input/output graph for the TK control (Figure 5-5, top right) looks similar to the graph showing the volume control effects for output compression (Figure 5-3, top left). This is because the TK control operates in a similar manner to the volume control for output compression hearing aids. On analog hearing aids, the TK control has been located at the input stage of the hearing aid (recall that in analog hearing aids the VC for output compression is positioned before the compressor and amplifier). It thus affects the amount of input signal that arrives at the compressor of the circuit, just like the VC does for output compression hearing aids.

It is very important to note that the left-most gain line, where there is greatest gain, shows the TK set to the *lowest* kneepoint position. The right-most gain line, where there is the least amount of gain, shows the TK set to the *highest* kneepoint position. As the compression kneepoint with the TK control is lowered, the gain for low-intensity input sounds is *increased*. Similarly, as the compression kneepoint with the TK control is raised, the gain for low-intensity input sounds is decreased.

When *listening* to a hearing aid with a TK control, it is important to let just the ambient noise of the room into the microphone in order to hear the effect of turning the control. With any input greater than the compression kneepoint (set by the TK control), the effect of adjusting the TK will not be audible. This is very different from the output limiting compression control where loud input sound becomes louder to the listener as the kneepoint is raised and the MPO is increased.

Clinical Uses of Output Linking and TK Compression Controls

Because the output linking compression control affects the MPO and not the gain, it can be used to limit the MPO to protect the client who wears the hearing aid from further hair cell damage and hearing loss. This type of compression control is especially useful for those clients who have a severe or profound hearing loss and a limited dynamic range. The output limiting type of compression control can be adjusted so that it limits the MPO of the hearing aid to a level that corresponds to the client's loudness tolerance levels. Some clinicians opt to set the MPO (measured in dB SPL) to be about 15 dB higher than the client's reported loudness tolerance levels (measured in dB HL). The rationale here is that the difference in dB HL versus dB SPL is close to an average of about 15 dB for the speech frequencies. As mentioned earlier, the output limiting compression control is most often found on *output* compression hearing aids, which are also more suited for severe-to-profound hearing loss.

As mentioned before, the TK control was initially associated with the KAmp™, which was a specific type of input compression hearing aid; namely, WDRC. This is discussed in further detail in the next section. The purpose behind the TK control is an attempt to imitate the function of the outer hair cells of the cochlea (Killion, 1996). In Chapter 1, it was mentioned that the outer hair cells amplify soft sounds (approximately less than 40 to 50 dB SPL) so that the inner hair cells can sense them. Use of the TK control is therefore most appropriate for mild-to-moderate SNHL. There is no real rule for adjusting the TK control; after all, what rule would one use to determine whether to adjust the TK control to say, 40 dB SPL versus 60 dB SPL inputs? The main reason the TK is adjustable in the first place, is to reduce the gain for quiet incoming sounds. A TK setting for maximum gain in quiet (e.g., the kneepoint set at 40 dB SPL) environments could result in the client being able to hear the internal amplifier and microphone noise of the hearing aid itself. The audible hiss can be annoying, especially for the client who has excellent low-frequency hearing. In general, raising the kneepoint setting of TK control so as to reduce the gain for very soft input sounds is not an issue for the client who presents with a flat, moderate SNHL. In today's digital hearing aids, "expansion" is commonly used along with the TK control, in order to reduce the audibility of the "hissing" sounds in quiet. More will be describe about expansion in Chapter 7.

Let's summarize where we have come so far. Four input/output graphs are shown in Figure 5–6. The top and bottom graphs on the left side fit together well; they both describe the two aspects of compression we have discussed so far, which are often combined on high-power hearing aids. The top-left graph shows the VC effects found on output compression; the client can adjust the gain by means of the VC, without any worries about affecting the MPO. The bottom-left graph shows the MPO adjustments that can be made by the hearing health care professional, based on the client's loudness tolerance. Together, on high-power hearing aids, these gain and MPO adjustments work well as a team.

The two graphs on the right show a combination of two compression characteristics that are commonly found together on moderate-power hearing aids. The top-right graph shows that with the VC, the client adjusts both the gain and MPO simultaneously. This is a satisfactory characteristic for moderate-power hearing aids because these cannot normally produce sufficient MPO that could further damage one's hearing. The bottom-right graph shows the effects of the TK control, which, like the output limiting compression control, is set by the health care professional. Many clinicians have been confused by the TK control and how it works. Again, it is very important to note that the left-most gain line, where there is greatest gain, shows the TK set to the *lowest* kneepoint position. The right-most gain line, where there is the least amount of gain, shows the TK set to the *highest* kneepoint position. As the compression kneepoint is lowered, the gain for low-intensity input sounds is increased! Similarly, as the kneepoint is raised, the gain for low-intensity input sounds is decreased. The general rule for setting the TK control is to set it as low as possible, in order to provide as much gain for soft incoming sounds as possible. Theoretically, the hearing aid would thus imitate the role of the outer hair cells.

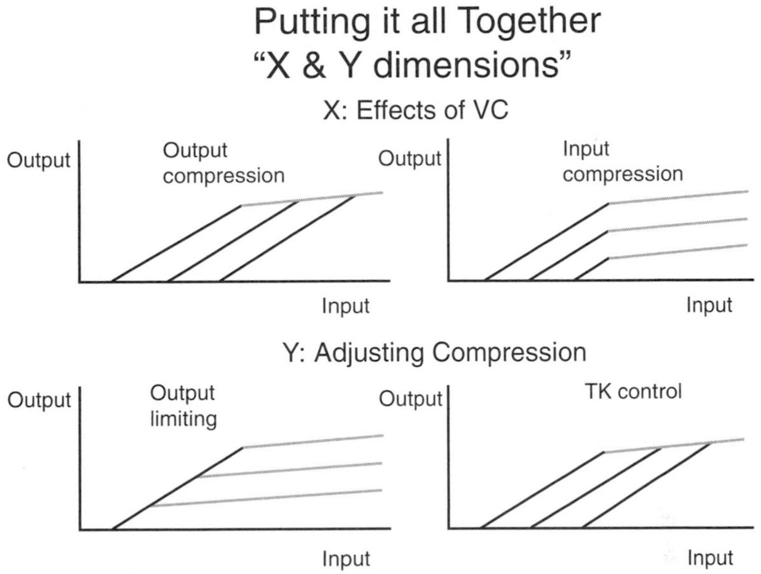

Putting it all Together
"X & Y dimensions"
X: Effects of VC

Y: Adjusting Compression

FIGURE 5–6 A summary of (1) input versus output compression and (2) output limiting compression control versus TK control is shown here. The volume control effects for input versus output compression can be seen on the top two graphs, while the effects of the different compression controls are displayed on the bottom two graphs. Most often, for severe-to-profound hearing loss, output compression is associated with the output limiting compression control (left-hand graphs). For mild-to-moderate SNHL, input compression is often associated with the TK control (right-hand graphs).

Lastly, note that the bottom-right graph for the TK control looks similar to the top-left graph showing the VC effects for output compression. On the older analog hearing aids, the TK control, like the VC on output compression hearing aids, was positioned before the compressor and amplifier. It thus operated in a similar manner to the VC for output compression hearing aids, by changing the amount of input signal that arrives at the compressor of the circuit. This is exactly what the VC did in the older analog hearing aids with output compression. With digital hearing aids, of course, all of these characteristics are achieved by means of mathematical software algorithms.

OUTPUT LIMITING COMPRESSION VERSUS WIDE DYNAMIC RANGE COMPRESSION (WDRC)

Two faces of compression have been discussed: (1) input versus output compression, and (2) the output limiting compression control versus the TK control. We now encounter the third, and last face of compression, which concludes our tour around the "sculpture" of compression. This "Z" dimension concerns "output limiting" compression versus "wide dynamic range" compression (WDRC), which

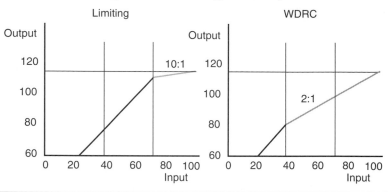

Output Limiting
versus
Wide Dynamic Range Compression

FIGURE 5–7   Input/output graphs also show effects of output limiting compression (left) and wide dynamic range compression (right). For both graphs, the diagonal lines rising from the X axis represent the gain; the corners represent the threshold kneepoint of compression; the lines to the right of the kneepoint represent the MPO. The hearing aid gain is the same (60 dB) for each type of compression. The gain function, however, is very different for each type of compression. Output limiting compression has a high kneepoint and a high compression ratio; linear (maximum) gain is provided for soft to medium input levels, and a high degree of compression suddenly limits the MPO. The focus of this compression combination is to "limit the ceiling" of loudness tolerance. WDRC has a low kneepoint and a low compression ratio; linear (maximum) gain takes place only for very soft inputs, while a weak degree of compression occurs for medium to intense input levels. The focus of this compression combination is to "lift the floor" of hearing sensitivity.

are really, two different compression schemes—they do not concern specific controls. Each of these compression schemes refers to separate ranges of compression threshold kneepoints, and compression ratios. The effects of output limiting compression and WDRC can be seen in Figure 5-7. Once again, both graphs in the figure are input/output graphs, similar to those in Figure 5-3 and 5-4.

Output Limiting Compression

Output limiting compression is typically associated with *output* compression hearing aids that use an output limiting compression control. As such, these three properties together are associated with high-power hearing aids for severe-to-profound SNHL. We have already mentioned that older analog hearing aids with input compression, utilized the output limiting compression control instead of the TK control; these same hearing aids also utilized output limiting compression. Let's look at output compression and see how it differs from WDRC.

The salient features of output limiting compression are shown in the left-most graph of Figure 5-7. Output limiting compression is associated with *"high"* compression kneepoints and *high* compression ratios. A high kneepoint means that the hearing aid begins to compress at relatively high input SPLs (i.e., 60 dB SPL or more). Below the kneepoint, the hearing aid provides linear gain.

We have already mentioned that compression ratios are the amount of compression provided by the hearing aid once compression begins. Recall that compression ratios can be visualized on an input/output graph by the slant of the line after (to the right of) the kneepoint. A 10:1 compression ratio is almost horizontal compared to that of a 2:1 ratio. Always remember that compression implies less gain than linear gain. A high compression ratio is usually defined as being greater than 4:1 (Venema, 2000). Higher compression ratios indicate *more* compression.

Output limiting compression hearing aids have a high kneepoint and a high ratio of compression. They provide a strong degree of compression over a narrow range of inputs (Figure 5-7, left graph). Below the threshold kneepoint, the output limiting compression hearing aid provides linear gain for a wide range of input SPLs. In other words, it "waits" for a fairly high input SPL to go into compression, but once it goes into compression, it *really* goes into compression.

Output limiting compression hearing aids have some similarities to linear hearing aids. They both give a fixed amount of gain over a wide range of different input SPLs, and then they both "suddenly" limit the output SPL. As mentioned earlier, the main difference between them is that linear hearing aids use peak clipping to limit the output, and output limiting compression hearing aids use a high ratio of compression to limit the output. The advantage of limiting the MPO with compression is that it introduces less distortion than peak clipping.

Wide Dynamic Range Compression (WDRC)

WDRC hearing aids became extremely popular during the 1990s. It is important to categorize where WDRC properly fits in the overall spectrum of the many faces of compression, because then, it can be appreciated for what it is, and what it is not.

WDRC is shown in Figure 5-7 (right graph). The TK control is used to adjust WDRC and like the TK control, WDRC has always been associated with *input* compression hearing aids. Recall, however, that not all input compression was WDRC; some analog input compression hearing aids used output limiting compression, which was adjusted by a conventional compression control. When teaching classes in hearing aid compression, the author often referred to these as the "odd ball" hearing aids, because they offered two ways to change the MPO: The VC as well as the output limiting compression control. Today, of course, these analog hearing aids have long since left the stage.

WDRC is associated with *low* threshold kneepoints (below 60 dB SPL) and *low* compression ratios (less than 4:1). As the right-most graph of Figure 5-7 shows, the WDRC hearing aid is almost always in compression, because all kinds of inputs, from very soft speech to a scream, will cause it to go into compression. Perhaps it was called "wide dynamic range compression" because of its low kneepoint, which allows compression to take place over a wide range of input intensity levels.

Once the WDRC hearing aid goes into compression, however, it does not provide a great ratio or degree of compression (Figure 5–7). Basically, a WDRC hearing aid provides a weak degree of compression over a wide range of inputs. The effect of WDRC is very different from output limiting compression or the old linear hearing aids, for that matter. Unlike those hearing aids that suddenly reduce the gain once the input SPL exceeds a certain amount, WDRC gradually reduces the gain for a wide range of input SPLs.

Clinical Applications of Output Limiting Compression and WDRC

When comparing output limiting compression with WDRC, it may be most useful and helpful to look closely at their names. The main clinical difference between the two is that output limiting compression does its work above its kneepoint; it reduces or limits the output for high input SPLs. On the other hand, WDRC does its work *below* its kneepoint; it increases its gain for sounds below the kneepoint by providing most (linear) gain for soft input sounds (Johnson, 1993; Killion, 1996).

Why would clinicians desire a choice between these two types of compression? To answer this question, it may be a good idea to take another look at loudness growth, already discussed in Chapter 4. The client who has outer hair cell damage usually has mild-to-moderate SNHL. For this person, the "floor" of hearing sensitivity is elevated compared to normal, although the "ceiling" of loudness tolerance is similar to normal. The appropriate goal of amplification is to restore normal loudness growth and to accomplish this goal, we need to amplify soft sounds by a lot, and loud sounds by little or nothing at all.

Here is some food for thought: It is no coincidence that, on the one hand, the KAmp™, WDRC, and on the other, oto-acoustic emissions and the knowledge of the role of the outer hair cells, became clinically popular at around the same time—the late 1980s and early 1990s.

Figure 5–8 shows output limiting compression (left) and WDRC (right) superimposed on two identical loudness growth graphs. Both graphs are the same as that of Figure 4–1, which shows the loudness growth functions of someone with normal hearing compared to that of someone with mild-to-moderate SNHL.

Figure 5–8 shows that both output limiting compression and WDRC may do the same thing for inputs of 100 dB; they may both reach the point where output sounds are perceived as being "too loud," but the *way* that each type of compression arrives at this common point is completely different. The author once attended an American Academy of Audiology conference seminar on compression given by F. Kuk back in 1996, who provided a very illustrative analogy. Output limiting compression was compared to a teenager speeding down the road in a relative's car who sees a stop sign at the end of the road and slams on the brakes and screeches to a stop. WDRC was compared to an elderly person who starts out at a normal speed, but on seeing the stop sign far ahead, ever so

Loudness Growth
&
Types of Compression

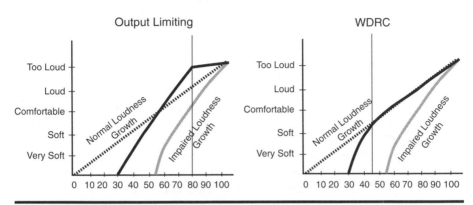

FIGURE 5–8   For mild-to-moderate SNHL, which is most common, re-establishing normal loudness growth is more easily achieved with WDRC than with output limiting compression. In both graphs, the X axis represents the physical dimension of input sound intensity to the hearing aid; the Y axis represents the psychoacoustic dimension of loudness perception (similar to Figure 4–1). In this example, both output limiting compression and wide dynamic range compression make 100 dB inputs sound "too loud." But the high kneepoint and high compression ratio for output limiting compression, make inputs of 80, 90, and 100 dB all sound "too loud" as well. This does not occur for WDRC, because it has a low kneepoint and a low compression ratio.

cautiously applies a foot gently to the brakes and slows to a stop over a long distance.

In the above analogy, normal loudness growth is the road. Some problems occur when trying to restore normal loudness growth with output limiting compression (Figure 5-8 left-most graph). First, there is an "overshoot" of normal loudness growth. The worst problem, however, is that amplified 70, 80, and 90 dB inputs all sound the same and are perceived as being "too loud." This does not restore normal loudness growth. The right-most graph shows WDRC applied to the same goal of restoring normal loudness growth. If restoring loudness growth is the goal, then the lower kneepoint and lower compression ratio that are provided by WDRC are clearly a much better fit, because soft sounds are perceived as louder, while loud sounds do not exceed the listener's comfort levels.

Maybe another reason for the term "WDRC" is that the low kneepoint and low compression ratio reduce a normally large dynamic range into the smaller one associated with mild-to-moderate SNHL. For example, a low compression ratio of 2:1 will compress a dynamic range of 100 dB into one of 50 dB.

Does this mean that all those with mild—moderate SNHL should "drive like the elderly person?" Not really. A client with mild—moderate SNHL may have become accustomed to wearing linear hearing aids with peak clipping, or those that provide linear gain and limit the MPO with output limiting compression. For this client, a sudden switch to WDRC might be too big a jump, and WDRC might be rejected because it is not "loud" enough. Although WDRC will amplify soft input SPLs by a lot, it will not amplify average intensity input SPLs by the same amount, and it is *this* difference that the client accustomed to linear amplification may find frustrating. Output limiting compression may result in the "overshoot" of normal loudness growth as seen in the left graph of Figure 5–8, but the client may have become accustomed to the sound. In this case, WDRC must be introduced gradually and with considerable counseling about what to expect from the hearing aids. Many such clients can adjust to WDRC, but others cannot seem to let go of their need for more power and refuse to make the change.

For the client with severe-to-profound hearing loss, output limiting compression might be a better choice than WDRC. These clients might prefer a strong, linear gain over a wide range of input SPLs, at least until the output SPL becomes close to their loudness tolerance or uncomfortable loudness levels. Furthermore, these clients often have worn this kind hearing aids in the past. High-power output limiting compression hearing aids will give lots of gain for soft sounds and the same "lots of gain" for average input sounds, such as speech, making it quite audible.

It should be appreciated that output limiting compression hearing aids have similar gain characteristics as linear hearing aids; they both provide linear gain over a wide range of soft to moderately intense input levels. More will be discussed about this similarity near the end of this chapter. In general, these two types of hearing aids do differ in one significant way: Instead of using peak clipping to limit the MPO, as the old linear hearing aids did, output limiting compression hearing aids offer a high degree of compression to accomplish the same thing. This introduces a lot less distortion than peak clipping.

It must be said here that hearing aids which provide linear gain can sound very "clean" and clear. This is because there is no compression taking place, which *can* audibly distort the sound quality. Linear gain can sound quite pleasing, as long as the input plus the gain does not *saturate* the hearing aid or, in other words, add up to equal the MPO. In short, output limiting compression may definitely be preferred by clients with severe-to-profound hearing loss.

WDRC can also be described in terms of its affect on the frequency response (Figure 5–9), much like we did with input versus output compression (Figure 5–4). Here it becomes quite evident that the gain of a WDRC hearing aid is highly dependent upon the input SPL, over a wide variety of input levels. In contrast to output limiting compression, where the gain reduces abruptly once a higher input sound level reaches the hearing aid, WDRC acts like a "trampoline"; its gain fluctuates with any input sound levels above its low kneepoint. Due to this phenomenon, WDRC is sometimes called "input level dependent compression."

WDRC: Displayed as a Frequency Response

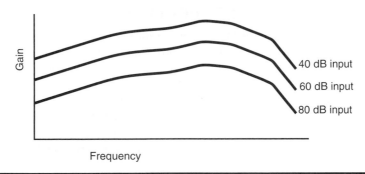

FIGURE 5–9 The effects of WDRC can also be seen on a frequency response, with varying input intensities. While the volume control is set to a typical preferred level, WDRC provides very different amounts of gain for widely ranging input intensities. These differences in gain for the same inputs, would not be apparent with output limiting compression; the same amounts of gain would be provided for the 40 and 60 dB SPL inputs. In other words, the two functions would be the same (or identical).

It has been suggested that the use of WDRC, along with fast attack/release times can degrade some of the cues necessary for speech recognition (Kuk, 1999). The reasoning is that, although WDRC amplifies soft speech more than loud speech, its use with fast attack/release times can reduce the differences between the "peaks" and "valleys" of the input speech sound wave. More on this topic is discussed in the section on "Syllabic Compression" later on in this chapter, and also, in Chapter 7.

For the purpose of sticking to clear definitions, a hearing aid with plain WDRC would tend to offer a fairly similar degree of compression across the frequencies. This is shown in Figure 5-9, where the difference in gain for each of the various input levels is consistent across the frequency response of the hearing aid. In the 1990s, some analog hearing aids with WDRC did exactly that. On those hearing aids, the low or high frequency gain could be adjusted with trimmers (either physical trimmers on the hearing itself or programmable trimmers), and such adjustments would result in an *equal* gain reduction for for all input levels, For example, to fit someone with a sloping high-frequency hearing loss, the clinician would cut some of the low-frequency gain. In Figure 5-9, this would be seen as an equal drop in all three lines on the graph, across the low frequencies.

The reason the point of equal amount of WDRC applied across the frequencies is highlighted here and also in Figure 5-9 is to point out how WDRC can also be specifically applied more at some frequencies than at others. This is explained further in the next section.

BILL AND TILL: TWO TYPES OF WDRC

Bass increase at low levels (BILL) and treble increases at low levels (TILL) are two types or subsets of WDRC. There are other names that pertain to these categories, such as LDFR (level-dependent frequency response), FDC (frequency-dependent compression), and ASP (automatic signal processing). Basically, these terms all boil down to at least one similar thing; namely, compression occurs more in some frequencies than in other frequencies. Where compression occurs, it will be WDRC, with a low kneepoint and a low compression ratio. The simplest classification of these types of compression is that of BILL and TILL (Killion, Staab, & Preves, 1990).

The advent of BILL took place in the mid 1980s; TILL came along with the analog KAmp™ circuit, developed by Killion, around 1989. So BILL is a bit older than TILL. BILL first appeared in a circuit known as the "Manhattan" circuit, created by the now-swallowed up company called "Argosy." It was called the Manhattan circuit because in a long-ago naming contest at the American Speech-Hearing Association, someone said its circuit board looked like the skyline of Manhattan. In subsequent circuits using BILL, it was also sometimes referred to as "automatic signal processing" (ASP).

Basically, BILL is WDRC confined to the bass frequencies, and TILL is WDRC confined to the treble frequencies. In any compression hearing aid, the compression kneepoint is often set at somewhat different input SPLs for different frequencies. Hearing aid specs sheets in North America don't show this; rather, they show the compression kneepoint on input/output graphs at 2000 Hz only. The reason is because 2000 Hz is a very important frequency required for the recognition of audible speech.

BILL and TILL, are unique hearing aids, in that the compression occurs at *very* different input SPLs for different frequencies. BILL hearing aids have a low kneepoint for the low frequencies and a higher kneepoint for the high frequencies. Low-frequency input will not have to be very intense to set the BILL hearing aid into compression, but high-frequency input will have to be much more intense to cause compression. This means that the BILL circuit will go into compression very often with low-frequency inputs, and not as often with high-frequency inputs Figure 5–10). BILL is basically WDRC occurring mainly in the low frequencies.

Figure 5–10 shows a simple set of gain and frequency graphs for BILL (left graph) and TILL (right graph) circuits. The BILL hearing aid (left graph) has a very broad or flat frequency response with soft inputs (e.g., 40 dB SPL). If input sound is produced so that it is at 40 dB SPL all across the frequency range, then the gain and frequency response of the BILL hearing aid will look something like the top flat line on the graph. As the input across frequencies is increased in intensity to 60 dB SPL, the gain and frequency response will reveal a decrease in

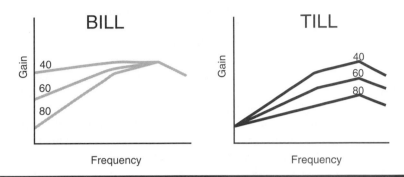

BILL & TILL
Two Types of WDRC

FIGURE 5–10   For each graph, the gain (Y axis) across a frequency range (X axis) is shown for three different input levels. The left graph shows BILL. As inputs decrease in intensity, low-frequency gain increases. Note that WDRC takes place only at the low frequencies, where the line functions are furthest apart. The right graph shows TILL. As inputs decrease in intensity, high-frequency gain increases. Again, WDRC here only takes place at the higher frequencies. This is evident because the lines are furthest apart at the high frequencies.

gain for the low frequencies. As the input intensity is increased to 80 dB SPL, the gain for the low frequencies will drop even more.

The main idea behind the BILL circuit is to enable better listening for speech while in background noise. That is, the "hubbub" of low-frequency background noise will be suppressed by compression, with the high-frequency sounds that render clarity for speech still receiving a full measure of gain. Again, the very different amounts of compression offered across the different frequencies underscores or emphasizes this fact. For these hearing aids (BILL and TILL), the input-output functions will look very different at different frequencies. As mentioned earlier, BILL first appeared in the "Manhattan" circuit; in the mid 1990s, Oticon took the concept of BILL and utilized it in the analog two-channel Multi-Focus™ hearing aid in 1995 (more on multi-channel hearing aids will be covered in Chapter 6). Later on, in 1997, Oticon again championed BILL in its first digital product, the DigiFocus™ (more will be covered on the topic of digital signal processing in Chapter 7). Oticon's stated purpose was to reduce the upward spread of masking. Recall from the earlier discussion on cochlear physiology in Chapter 1, this phenomenon refers to the fact that low frequencies mask high frequencies better than highs mask lows. BILL was seen as a way to fight the upward spread of masking, so as to increase speech intelligibility in background noise.

The TILL hearing aid (right graph) is completely different. The original analog TILL hearing aids were those that utilized the K Amp™ circuit. These hearing aids first appeared around 1989, and quickly became extremely popular. The kneepoint is set at a low input level for the high frequencies. For the TILL hearing aid, high-frequency input will not have to be very intense to cause compression. This means the TILL circuit will go into compression very often with high-frequency inputs, and not as often with low-frequency inputs. TILL is basically WDRC confined to the high frequencies.

Figure 5–10 (right graph) shows a TILL response. For the TILL hearing aid, low-intensity input SPLs of 40 dB across the frequency range will result in a gain and frequency response that has more of a high-frequency emphasis. As the input is increased to 60 dB SPL, the high-frequency emphasis will decrease relative to the gain for the low frequencies. With inputs of 80 dB SPL, the gain for the high frequencies will decrease even more. In some TILL in-the-ear hearing aids, the 80 plus dB SPL response was intended to resemble the resonance of the open, unaided ear, thus providing an acoustic "transparency" for intense inputs when amplification is not needed.

The main idea behind TILL is to emphasize the high-frequency sounds of speech for the listener who most typically has high-frequency hearing loss. As discussed in Chapter 4, this client will have a reduced dynamic range for the high frequencies. Compared to that for normal hearing, the "floor" of hearing sensitivity will be elevated, although the "ceiling" of loudness tolerance will not be.

COMMON CLINICAL COMBINATIONS OF COMPRESSION

Let's summarize where we have come so far. Three dimensions of compression were woven together in Chapter 4: (1) output versus input compression, (2) output limiting compression controls versus the TK control, and (3) output limiting compression versus WDRC. The six static aspects of compression are often found together in two common compression combinations, and each combination can serve a different clinical population (Figure 5–11). Although there are no absolute maxims for endorsing one type of compression over another, there are, however, some trends, as described here. It reinforced here yet again, that an appreciation of these combinations of compression, as they first appeared in analog hearing aids is essential in order to understand today's digital hearing aid technology.

A Compression Combination for Severe-to-Profound Hearing Loss

Output compression, output limiting compression, along with the use of an output limiting compression control work well together in the same circuit. This combination has several features for clients with severe-to-profound hearing loss, which usually results in a small dynamic range (i.e., about 20 dB). With high-power hearing aids, protection of residual hearing is critical for these clients. Using output compression, the client can be assured that although the VCs of these hearing aids change the kneepoint of compression, they affect only the

Summary:
Applying Compression

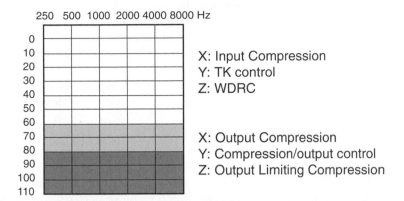

250 500 1000 2000 4000 8000 Hz

X: Input Compression
Y: TK control
Z: WDRC

X: Output Compression
Y: Compression/output control
Z: Output Limiting Compression

FIGURE 5–11   WDRC, which is a type of input compression that utilizes the TK control, is well suited for fitting mild-to-moderate SNHL. Output limiting, which is almost always used with output compression circuits, and which is adjusted with an output limiting control, is suited for fitting severe-to-profound hearing losses. The shaded area in the range from 60 to 80 dB hearing losses, represents a "gray" area of intersection for the fitting of either type of compression.

gain and *not* the MPO. Independent from the VC, a conventional compression control in the hearing aid also changes the compression kneepoint, and this adjusts the MPO (see also Figure 5-6). Specifically, as the kneepoint is *raised*, the MPO is also *raised*. The output limiting compression in the hearing aid means that the compression kneepoint occurs at a relatively high input level, along with a high ratio or degree of compression. If the hearing aid has a high-power circuit, the client receives lots of linear gain for soft to at least conversational speech input levels, but once the output comes close to the individual's loudness tolerance levels, the hearing aid suddenly provides a high degree of compression, so as to limit the output. Although normal loudness growth is not been achieved for these clients, they do get a strong degree of amplification along with a limited maximum output.

A Compression Combination for Mild-to-Moderate Hearing Loss

Input compression, WDRC, along with the use of a TK control also work well together in the same circuit (Figure 5-11). This combination has several features that address the needs of clients with mild-to-moderate SNHL, which usually results in a dynamic range of at least 40 dB to 60 dB. With input compression, the VC does not affect the kneepoint of compression, but it does affect the gain and the MPO together. A TK control changes the kneepoint of compression, and it also specifically affects the gain for soft incoming sounds (see also Figure 5–6). Recall that the TK control does not affect the gain for loud inputs. Specifically, as the kneepoint is *lowered*, the gain for soft inputs is *increased*. The WDRC in the hearing aid means that the kneepoint of compression occurs at a relatively low input level, along with a low ratio or degree of compression. WDRC hearing aids usually have a medium-power circuit, which means the client receives linear gain for only very soft input levels. The hearing aid is otherwise in a low degree of compression over a wide range of medium to intense input levels. With these features, clients get a greater degree of amplification for soft input sounds and less amplification for sounds that are well within their dynamic range.

Recall from Chapters 2 and 3 that for clients with mild-to-moderate SNHL, the cochlear damage most often concerns the outer hair cells. As a result, the "floor" of hearing sensitivity is raised, while the "ceiling" of loudness tolerance may be quite similar to that of normal hearing. Input compression with WDRC is applicable to the largest clinical population (i.e., those persons with mild-to-moderate SNHL). It is, therefore, very important to categorize the increasingly popular types of input compression (Figure 5–12).

A visual categorization of input compression is shown in Figure 5–12. As the philosopher John Quine once said, "Categorization is the essence of intelligence." First, look at the outside ring of the circle shown in the figure. This represents the historical development of input compression that was not WDRC. These were often high-power, analog input compression hearing aids hearing aids that have a conventional output limiting compression control that adjusts the MPO; they also utilize output limiting compression, which consists of a high kneepoint and a high compression ratio. In the author's opinion, input compression that is not WDRC was an "oddball" combination of compression characteristics, a "department of redundancy department," because they offered two ways of adjusting the MPO: the VC adjusts it as well as the compression control!

On the other hand, WDRC is *always* found along with input compression. WDRC is a type of input compression, but not all input compression is WDRC. Similarly, BILL and TILL are two types of WDRC, but not all WDRC is specifically BILL or TILL. The analog K Amp^{TM} hearing aid circuit of the 1990s was TILL, a type of WDRC, which in turn is also a type of input compression. The analog Oticon Multifocus^{TM} hearing aid, also of the 1990s, was BILL, another type of WDRC. Recall that BILL hearing aids offer most compression for the low frequencies and TILL offers most compression for the high frequencies. A straight WDRC hearing aid that is neither BILL nor TILL offers a more similar degree of compression across the frequencies. *Today's digital hearing aids readily and commonly utilize all types of compression mentioned so far.*

Now let's place all the hearing aids we have discussed together, next to each other, on a clinical "spectrum" (Figure 5–13): the old linear gain hearing aid with peak clipping, the newer hearing aids that began to offer output limiting compression (which first appeared in the late 1970s), and the newer still hearing aids that offered WDRC (which first appeared in the 1980s). Linear peak

Categorizing AGCi, WDRC, BILL & TILL

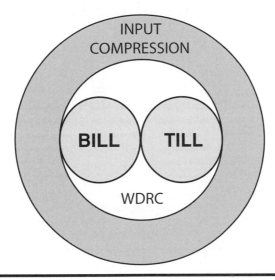

FIGURE 5–12   Because input compression can be applied to a large segment of the hearing aid fitting population, input compression is most widely used. For analog hearing aids of the past, which provided only one type of compression or another, input compression had the most subdivisions. Clinicians thus found some categorization helpful. As shown, all WDRC is input compression, but not all input compression is WDRC. Furthermore, BILL and TILL are WDRC, but not all WDRC is BILL or TILL. This is because input compression that is not WDRC (outer circle) has compression kneepoints and ratios that are more like those of output limiting compression. Some WDRC is neither BILL nor TILL; in this case, low inputs result in an equal amount of gain increase at all frequencies, as was shown in Figure 5-9.

clipping hearing aids are more similar or closer in relationship to output limiting compression hearing aids than they are to WDRC hearing aids. Thus, output limiting is like a bridge between linear peak clipping and WDRC. At the risk of repetition, it is worth repeating a point earlier: Output limiting "does its work" above its threshold kneepoint to limit the output, while WDRC "does its work" below its kneepoint to increase the gain for soft sounds.

   Linear hearing aids once enjoyed a wide but diminishing range of fitting applicability; they were routinely fit on the majority of clients up until as recently as the late 1980s! Linear circuitry can provide a lot of gain for severe-to-profound hearing losses or less gain for mild-to-moderate hearing losses. Their most salient feature is that they give the same gain for all input levels. Note on the left-most graphic of Figure 5-13, that soft, average, and loud inputs are all "elevated" by the same amount. The worst thing about this linear type of gain is that the MPO is limited with peak clipping. Sound that is limited in this manner is often distorted and has poor quality for the listener.

Summary
A Clinical "Spectrum" of Hearing Aids

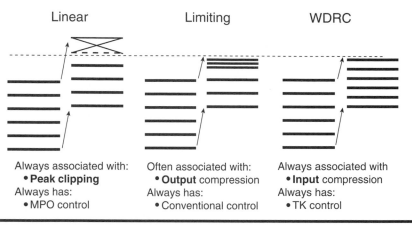

Linear   Limiting   WDRC

Always associated with: Often associated with: Always associated with
• **Peak clipping**   • **Output** compression   • **Input** compression
Always has: Always has: Always has:
• MPO control   • Conventional control   • TK control

FIGURE 5–13   For each of three types of hearing aids shown here, two sets of horizontal lines and arrows are shown. The left lines represent the input, the arrows represent the gain, and the right lines represent the output. The dotted line represents the loudness tolerance level for some particular client. For linear hearing aids, the gain is the same for all input levels. When the output reaches the "ceiling" of loudness tolerance, the output is clipped, resulting in distortion of sound quality. For output limiting hearing aids, only the top "output" lines are squeezed together, because the gain is linear for soft and average input sound, and is dramatically reduced for high-intensity input sounds. For wide dynamic range compression hearing aids, both the input and output lines are evenly spread apart because the gain is gradually reduced as the input intensity increases. A large dynamic range is "evenly" shrunk into a smaller one, which restores normal loudness growth.

The output limiting compression hearing aid (usually found together with output compression) once represented compression in general. It was most often associated with high-power circuitry, however, which provides a lot of gain for the client with severe-to-profound hearing loss. As such, it serviced the needs of clients for whom loudness tolerance was a major concern. The middle graphic on Figure 5–13 shows that with its high kneepoint of compression and high compression ratio, the output limiting compression hearing aid "elevates" soft and average input levels by the same amount. In this way it was like the linear hearing aid on the left. Unlike the linear hearing aid, however, the output limiting compression hearing aid had an output limiting compression control that enabled compression (instead of peak clipping) to limit the output. This is accomplished without the degree of distortion often associated with linear peak clipping.

In the world of compression in analog hearing aids, WDRC was the "new kid on the block," first appearing in the late 1980s. As a type of input compression,

WDRC hearing aids often provided less gain than the output limiting hearing aid. The right-most graph on Figure 5-13 shows that with its low threshold knee-point and low compression ratio, the WDRC hearing aid gave progressively less and less gain as the inputs increase. Recall that the focus of WDRC is to restore normal loudness growth by shrinking a large dynamic range into a smaller one. The gain, however, does *not* decrease to the same degree as the input SPLs increase; otherwise the output would remain the *same* for all input levels. The gain must go down more slowly than the input SPLs go up.

When WDRC first appeared, experienced clinicians were fond of pointing out the difficulties of fitting WDRC hearing aids on clients who are accustomed to wearing linear hearing aids; these clients initially found that the WDRC hearing aids were "not loud enough." For soft input sounds, the WDRC hearing aids were satisfactory because it is for these sounds that they provided the most gain; however, with their low compression kneepoint and low ratio of compression, the WDRC circuit did not provide as much gain as the older linear hearing aids did for average-to-intense input sounds. A common clinical report was that clients who were accustomed to linear peak clipping, therefore, initially rejected WDRC. As a transition to WDRC from linear gain, it was suggested to fit them with output limiting compression, because this type of compression is closer to linear peak clipping. On the other hand, for new clients with mild-to-moderate SNHL who have never worn hearing aids before, WDRC may provide a very good fit.

DYNAMIC ASPECTS OF COMPRESSION

Until now, compression has been discussed in terms of threshold kneepoint and compression ratio. These are sometimes known as the "static" aspects of compression, because they involve the input SPL when compression begins and the degree of compression once it occurs. Sound in the environment, however, is constantly changing in intensity over time and a compression hearing aid has to respond to these changes in intensity over time. The "dynamic" aspects of compression are known as the "attack" and the "release" times.

The attack and release times are the lengths of time it takes for a compression circuit to respond to changes in the intensity of an input SPL (Figure 5-14). When the input SPL exceeds the kneepoint of compression, the hearing aid "attacks" the sound by reducing the gain. Once the input sound falls below the kneepoint of compression, the hearing aid "releases" from compression and restores the gain. The attack time is the length of time it takes for a hearing aid to go into compression and reduce the gain; the release time is the length of time it takes for it to come out of compression and restore the gain.

An electrical circuit cannot instantly mirror the changes that take place in the environment, because it requires time to respond to these changes. For example, if a compression circuit is to respond to a sudden input SPL increase, it has to wait for at least one cycle of the sound wave to "know" if the increased SPL will remain. A change in gain that occurs faster than the longest cycle or

Dynamic Compression Characteristics

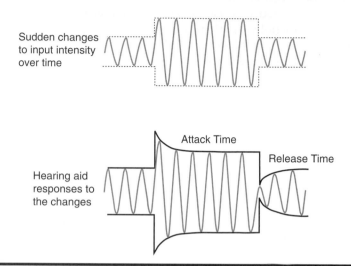

FIGURE 5–14 The top shows a simple description of input sound changing in intensity (vertical dimension) over time (horizontal dimension). The sound has suddenly increased in intensity and after a while the sound suddenly decreases in intensity. The bottom shows the output response of a compression hearing aid to the changes in sound input intensity over time. Note that gain has been applied to even the soft input, before the sudden intensity increase. The compression circuitry takes some amount of time to respond or compress the incoming signal that has suddenly increased in intensity. This is the "attack" time. Once the input sound has decreased in intensity, the circuit takes some time to stop compressing. This is the "release" time.

period of incoming sound can change the fine details of the sound waves and distortion will result.

Hearing aids are not the only electrical devices that use compression and have attack/release times. Audiovisual equipment has used input and output compression for many years and we have heard its effects before. Recall, for example, the television broadcasts in which the sports announcer is talking and the background noise is changing in intensity over time. When a score is made and the audience suddenly increases their cheers, the background noise increases in intensity. It may take a short time for the compression of the audiovisual equipment to attack and reduce the gain of the noise; but this also temporarily reduces the gain for the announcer's voice. When the cheering stops, it may again take some time for the system to release from compression; and the announcer's voice will accordingly take some time to return back to a normal, audible level.

Most attack and release times are set to achieve a best compromise between two undesirable extremes. Times that are too fast will cause the gain to fluctuate rapidly and this may cause a jarring, "pumping" perception by the listener. Times that are too slow may make the compression act too slowly and cause a real lagging perception on the part of the listener. Quick attack times (i.e., 10 ms or less) might prevent sudden, transient sounds from becoming too loud for the listener. In general, release times need to be longer than attack times to prevent a "fluttering" perception on the part of the listener (Staab, 1996). Longer release times (i.e., up to 150 ms) tend to prevent distortions that can occur with fast release times. Inordinately fast release times can cause the hearing aid to track the amplitude of individual cycles of sound waves (Staab, 1996). Such a rapid modulation of sound can cause a "breathing" or "pumping" perception on the part of the listener (Armstrong, 1996).

Just as we have seen with the static aspects of compression, there are lots of "buzz" words that float around when the dynamic aspects of compression are discussed. Different attack and release times are sometimes used to categorize different types of dynamic compression. Various types of dynamic compression methods are discussed briefly below.

Peak Detection

Most analog compression hearing aids have used a technique called peak detection to "track" the peak amplitude of incoming sound waves. If the peak is greater than the compression threshold kneepoint, the circuit attacks and begins to compress the signal, which reduces the gain. Once the peak is below the kneepoint, the compression releases and the gain increases again. Peak detection allowed for a wide variety of times that could separately be specified and assigned as attack and release times; however, these times were constant and fixed for any incoming sound intensity patterns (Armstrong, 1993). Most peak detection systems in hearing aids were adjusted to provide *quick* attack times and *longer, slower* release times.

An advantage of peak detection is that it reacts very quickly to increases in environmental sound levels. Unfortunately, however, it can react inappropriately to very short intense sounds, because the longer release times will keep the gain down after the short intense sound has stopped. This may unnecessarily reduce the gain of sounds the listener might want to hear.

With fixed attack/release times, the hearing aid cannot respond differently to different patterns of sound input intensities when needed. As discussed in Chapter 3, speech is an example of sound that is constantly changing over time. The dynamic acoustic sounds of speech within the world of ever-changing background noise (e.g., the sudden slamming of a door or the constant roar of traffic) can pose listening problems for the peak detection method and the listener.

"Syllabic compression" and "automatic volume control" (AVC) are two specific sets of attack/release times commonly encountered on today's digital hearing aids. In the past, some high-end analog hearing aids employed the use of either syllabic or AVC. Today, these attack/release time schemes, as well as those of average detection (described later on), can often be selected alternately on fitting software for digital hearing aids. The most high-profile usage of syllabic compression occurred with the advent of the Oticon DigiFocus™, in 1997.

Automatic Volume Control

A type of compression known as "automatic volume control" (AVC) has often been used during broadcasts with audiovisual equipment. In a comparison to peak detection, AVC has a relatively long attack and long release times; its release times are usually more than 150 ms and can be as long as several seconds (Hickson, 1994). Because of this, it does not respond to rapid fluctuations of sound input. On the contrary, it responds mainly to general, overall changes in sound intensity, which reduces the need for the listener to adjust the volume control manually. The long attack/release times with AVC are intended to imitate the length of time it physically takes for a listener to react to sudden noise increases by raising a hand and manually adjusting the VC on a hearing aid, hence, its name! The most high-profile usage of AVC occurred with the Widex Senso™ digital hearing aid in 1997. The Senso™ was the very first digital product to appear in BTE and ITE formats.

Syllabic Compression

"Syllabic compression" refers to the exact opposite of AVC; namely, relatively short attack and release times; its release times vary from less than 50 ms up to 150 ms. The attack/release times are specifically intended to be shorter than the duration of the typical speech syllable, which is about 200 to 300 ms (Hickson, 1994). Short attack/release times allow the hearing aid to compress or reduce the gain for the peaks of more intense speech (usually the vowel sounds), and this provides more uniformity in the intensity of ongoing speech syllables. In other words, syllabic compression reduces the differences between the normally more intense vowels and the softer unvoiced consonants such as /s/. The main premise of syllabic compression is to allow a hearing aid to make the softer sounds of speech more audible without simultaneously making the normally louder parts of speech from becoming too loud.

Syllabic compression is somewhat controversial and not everyone agrees with its use. Because syllabic compression compresses the peaks of speech and makes the waveform of ongoing speech more uniform, noise can easily fill in the small gaps that remain (Johnson, 1993), and in noisy situations, a hearing aid might amplify the noise that is situated between the peaks of speech. According to Killion (1996), fast attack/release times of 50 ms can distort the waveform of speech, and, thus, compromise speech intelligibility.

As mentioned in the earlier section in this chapter on WDRC, Kuk (1999) suggests that the use of fast attack/release times (less than 10 ms) and short release times (less than 100 ms) will compromise the intensity differences between the various phonetic elements of speech. Specifically, in the time waveform of speech, the differences between the "peaks" or loud elements and "valleys," or soft elements are compromised or lessoned by fast attack/release times. Such a reduction, in turn, can distort the spectral content of speech cues. It is interesting to note that the opposites of AVC and syllabic compression were used in the very first two digital hearing aids (Widex Senso™ and Oticon DigiFocus™), and continue to be used today. A firm conclusion has not been reached. Obviously, the jury is still out. More will be discussed on these two pioneers of digital hearing aids near the end of Chapter 7.

As mentioned earlier, in the mid to late 90s, Oticon promoted the use of syllabic compression along with BILL, in its analog Multi-Focus™ hearing aid and digital DigiFocus™ hearing aids, in order to improve aided speech recognition, by reducing the upward spread of masking. Oticon used syllabic compression in the low frequencies, along with a simultaneous use of BILL (as described earlier). Thus, not only was WDRC present especially for the low frequencies, but the WDRC was made to act quickly. If the normally loud, low-frequency background noise can be thought of as the bull, and relatively soft, high-frequency consonants as fragile china teacups, then syllabic compression used in conjunction with BILL could be a way to control the raging bull in the china shop.

Adaptive Compression™

This type of compression has fixed, quick attack times, but has release times that vary with the length or duration of the intense, incoming sound. For short (transient) intense sound inputs, the release time is short. For sound inputs that are longer in rise time and duration, the release times are longer. The desired result is a reduction of compression "pumping" heard by the listener. Adaptive compression™ was originally patented by Telex and then became most commonly associated with the KAmp™ circuits.

Average Detection

Average detection was first associated with the DynamEQII™ circuit by Gennum. This circuit was one of the original analog two-channel WDRC hearing aid circuits that emerged during the mid 1990s (following the two-channel circuit produced by ReSound). These multi-channel hearing aids commonly emerged with BILL being used in the low-frequency channel, and TILL being used in the high-frequency channel. More will be described on multi-channel hearing aids in Chapter 6. Unlike the peak detection method that tracks the peak amplitude of incoming sound waves, the average detection method looks at the average of incoming signal over a given length of time. When the average SPL exceeds the kneepoint of compression, then the gain is reduced. For the purpose of explaining the average detection, its historical implementation in the analog, two-channel DynamEQII™ will be explained below. It should, again, be realized that digital hearing aids utilize mathematical algorithms to accomplish similar results.

The analog DynamEQII™ had "twin" average compression detectors; one was a fast detector and the other was a slow detector (see Figure 5–15).

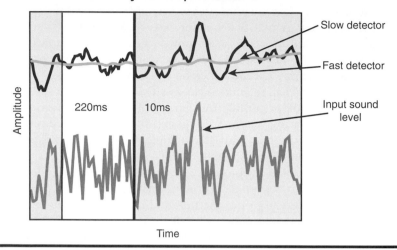

An Example of Slow and Fast Activity Compression

Slow detector

Fast detector

Input sound level

220ms   10ms

Amplitude

Time

FIGURE 5–15   The figure shows the actions of "average" detection. A slow average detector is often used in concert with a fast average detector. The slow detector averages sound over time intervals of about 220 ms, and the fast average detector averages sound over time intervals of about 10 ms. The bottom line represents sound intensity as it <u>occurs</u> over time. The top smooth line represents the input signal when averaged by the slow average detector. Note that the slow average is very flat over time. The top bumpy line represents the input signal when averaged by the fast detector. Note the fast average changes a lot more over time than the slow average. The net effect of this kind of system is that intense incoming transient sounds are given quick attack/release times, while incoming sounds that take longer to become intense and quiet again are given relatively longer attack/release times.

The slow average detector averaged sound inputs over a 220 ms time interval (i.e., about 1/5 of a second) and was in control of the compression system most of the time. When the slow average of incoming sounds exceeded the threshold kneepoint of compression, the gain was slowly reduced and was hardly noticeable. With the slow detector alone, however, a short spike of intense sound could be averaged into the overall body of sound taking place over 220 ms. This slow average would not be enough to "tell" the hearing aid to go into compression and reduce the gain. This is where the fast average detector came into the picture. The fast average detector averages sound inputs over time intervals of about 10 ms (i.e., 1/100 of a second) and it acted when intense transients were not "caught" by the slow detector. When the "fast" average was 6 dB greater than the "slow" average, the fast average detector took over and reduced the gain for the spike of intense sound.

The main result of average detection is that both the attack and release times vary with the length of the incoming intense sounds. This is in direct contrast to the peak detection systems that give constant, fixed quick attack and slow release times for all incoming stimuli. As long as the incoming sounds are below the compression threshold, both types of circuits provide uncompressed gain. With sudden transient loud sounds, however, such as a door slam, the average detection system will provide quick attack and quick release times. On the other hand, the peak detector will provide its usual quick attack and slow release times. Because of the reduction of gain and the long recovery of the peak detection circuit, soft speech spoken right after the door slam may be temporarily inaudible to the listener. The average detection circuit enables a quick recovery of gain after the door slam, because, its release time will be quick for short sounds.

The benefit to the listener is that there is less "pumping" perception. The average detection system is a compromise between compression that reacts to every short intense sound and compression that may react too slowly for some sounds that should be compressed. Audible by-products of compression should not become a nuisance to listeners. Dynamic aspects should be considered when trying to make hearing aids acoustically "transparent."

The various dynamic compression characteristics described above can be selected for most of today's digital hearing aids on the fitting software. For the most part, on most manufacturers' fitting software, the choice is largely between syllabic compression and average detection. Most often, syllabic compression is selected for the low-frequency channels of the digital hearing aid, and average detection is selected for the higher-frequency channels.

Recall that Widex promoted the use of AVC on its Senso™ digital hearing aid; the reason was because field trial subjects who first tried the Senso liked it best. Recall also that syllabic compression was utilized for the low frequencies on Oticon's DigiFocus™. There you have it; opposite attack/release time schemes for the first two small-sized digital hearing aids out in the marketplace. The jury is obviously out regarding the best attack/release times.

INTERACTION BETWEEN STATIC AND DYNAMIC ASPECTS OF COMPRESSION

Compression consists of static aspects in one dimension and dynamic aspects in a purely separate dimension. With incoming sounds, the attack/release times of a hearing aid interact with the ratio of compression (Armstrong, 1996). The input/output graphs on hearing aid spec sheets show compression ratios that are obtained with constant pure tones, not the stops and starts of sounds like speech. Static compression ratios on spec sheets do not accurately represent the actual compression ratios experienced in real life by clients who wear the hearing aids. Fast attack/release times have the effect of temporarily reducing the ratio or amount of compression for any given sound stimulus.

Attack and release times interact with compression ratios and these interactions affect the sound quality for the listener. In general, a combination of short attack/release times (e.g., 10 ms) and high compression ratios (e.g., 10:1) the greatest distortion. If the same short attack/release times are used with low compression ratios (e.g., 2:1), then the sound quality is not as distorted (Armstrong, 1996). On the other hand, long attack/release times can be combined with either high or low compression ratios.

Dynamic aspects and static aspects of compression are often found in predictable combinations today. Syllabic compression, with its relatively short attack and release times, is most often associated with WDRC hearing aids that have a low-compression kneepoint and a low-compression ratio of less than 5:1. It is less common with output limiting compression hearing aids where the kneepoints and ratios of compression are "high." AVC, with its relatively long attack/release times, is most often seen in hearing aids that offer a low-threshold kneepoint of compression and high-compression ratio (Hickson, 1994).

SUMMARY

- In this chapter, we have looked at some of the many faces of compression. With input/output graphs, compression was explored along three angles or dimensions: (X) input versus output compression, (Y) the conventional compression control versus the "TK" control, and (Z) output limiting compression versus WDRC.

- From a clinician's point of view, the main difference between input and output compression is the effect of the volume control. With output compression, the volume control affects the gain but not the MPO. With input compression, the volume control affects both the gain and the MPO.

- The effects of the output limiting control and the TK control were compared, with the VC held constant. The former compression control affects the threshold kneepoint of compression and also the MPO. The TK control affects the kneepoint and the gain for soft inputs only. The effect of the output limiting compression control is audible only when speaking loudly into the hearing aid; the effect of the TK control is audible only when speaking softly into the hearing aid.

- Output limiting compression was compared to WDRC regarding compression kneepoints and compression ratios. Output limiting compression has a high kneepoint, which means that compression is activated only for relatively intense sound input levels; it also has a high compression ratio. WDRC has a low kneepoint and a low compression ratio. These differences separate their respective clinical purposes. Output limiting acts mostly above its kneepoint to limit the output. WDRC acts mostly below its kneepoint to provide most gain for soft input sounds.

- Output compression is most often associated with output limiting compression and it is adjusted by an output limiting control. This combination can be very appropriate for severe-to-profound hearing loss that usually exhibits a narrow dynamic range. Input compression is often associated with WDRC, and it is adjusted with a TK control. This combination can be very appropriate for mild-to-moderate SNHL, which usually exhibits a wider dynamic range.

- Mild-to-moderate SNHL is very common and WDRC is also very popular. Two subsets of WDRC are BILL and TILL.

- Dynamic aspects of compression were discussed separately from the static compression aspects of compression threshold kneepoint and compression ratio. Different types of attack/release time parameters were discussed. The usual compromise has been to provide fast attack times with longer release times.

- AVC and syllabic compression were described as being opposites. AVC has long attack/release times, and syllabic compression offers relatively short attack/release times. AVC is chosen for client comfort; the attack/release times are intended to mimic the length of time it takes for someone to physically adjust the VC. Syllabic detection is chosen to reduce the upwards spread of masking. Adaptive compression offers fixed attack times and variable release times, while average detection offers variable attack and release times. Both adaptive and average detection are designed to reduce the adverse perception of audible hearing aid amplifier "pumping."

- The 1990s were the "golden" age of compression, because compression types flourished and differentiated, and yet, all hearing aids were still analog. This meant that each hearing aid was confined to providing one type of compression or another. In order to choose the appropriate hearing aid products for their clients, clinicians thus needed to understand each type of compression well, and categorize these among all available types of compression.

REVIEW QUESTIONS

1. The volume control on output compression (AGCo) hearing aids affects:
   a. gain, but not MPO.
   b. MPO but not gain.
   c. gain and MPO together.
   d. none of the above

2. The conventional compression control affects:
   a. MPO.
   b. gain for any input intensity level.
   c. gain for soft inputs only.
   d. none of the above

3. The TK control affects:
   a. MPO.
   b. gain for any input intensity level.
   c. gain for soft inputs only.
   d. none of the above

4. WDRC is associated with:
   a. high kneepoint and high compression ratio.
   b. low kneepoint and high compression ratio.
   c. high kneepoint and low compression ratio.
   d. low kneepoint and low compression ratio.

5. The following statement is true:
   a. All input compression is WDRC, but not all WDRC is input compression.
   b. All WDRC is input compression, but not all input compression is WDRC.
   c. All output compression is WDRC, but not all WDRC is output compression.
   d. All WDRC is output compression, but not all output compression is WDRC.

6. BILL and TILL are two types of:
   a. WDRC.
   b. output compression.
   c. compression controls.
   d. input limiting.

7. WDRC provides most gain for:
   a. soft input sounds .
   b. medium input sounds.
   c. loud input sounds.
   d. all of the above

8. To hear the effect of a TK compression control, you should:
   a. adjust the volume control and let only really soft sounds into the mic.
   b. adjust the volume control and talk loudly into the mic.
   c. turn the compression control and let only really soft input sounds into the mic.
   d. turn the compression control and talk loudly into the mic.

9. A compression control that changes the MPO is most often found on hearing aids with:
   a. output compression.
   b. input compression.
   c. WDRC.
   d. linear gain.

10. As you lower the kneepoint with an output limiting compression control, you:

    a. increase the MPO.

    b. decrease the MPO.

    c. decrease gain for soft inputs.

    d. increase gain for soft inputs.

11. For mild-moderate SNHL, the following three compression features are often found together:

    a. input compression, high kneepoint & ratio, TK control.

    b. output compression, high kneepoint & ratio, output limiting compression control.

    c. input compression, low kneepoint & ratio, TK control.

    d. output compression, low kneepoint & ratio, output limiting compression control.

12. For severe-profound HL, the following three compression features are often found together:

    a. input compression, high kneepoint & ratio, TK control.

    b. output compression, high kneepoint & ratio, output limiting compression control.

    c. input compression, low kneepoint & ratio, TK control.

    d. output compression, low kneepoint & ratio, output limiting compression control.

13. On input/output graphs, the left-most diagonal line represents the:

    a. least gain.

    b. least compression.

    c. most gain.

    d. highest kneepoint.

14. A compression hearing aid provides 90 dB output with 40 dB input; what's the gain here?

15. Same hearing aid: kneepoint at 50 dB SPL, compression ratio of 2:1; the output for a 60 dB input is:

16. Same hearing aid: kneepoint at 50 dB SPL, compression ratio of 2:1; the gain for a 60 dB input is:

17. A compression hearing aid provides 120dB output with 50 dB input; what's the gain here?

18. Same hearing aid: kneepoint at 70 dB SPL, compression ratio of 10:1; the output for an 80 dB input is:

19. Same hearing aid: kneepoint at 70 dB SPL, compression ratio of 10:1; the output for a 90 dB input is:

20. You are fitting a hearing aid; the kneepoint is 40 dB SPL and the compression ratio is 2:1. Your probe tube mic (real-ear) system does not work well for inputs below 50 dB SPL. From the output for a 50 dB SPL input, the calculated gain is 30 dB. What would the gain be if you ran a curve using a 40 dB SPL input? Hint: an I/O graph can really help to figure it out.

RECOMMENDED READINGS

Compression handbook: An overview of the characteristics and applications of compression amplification. 1996 Eden Prairie, MN: Starkey Marketing Services, Starkey Labs, Inc., 1996.

Killion, M. C. (1997). A critique on four popular statements about compression. *The Hearing Review, 4*(2), 36–56.

REFERENCES

Armstrong, S. (1996, September). *Chips and dips-an engineering perspective of hearing aid circuits, power supplies, and the like.* Paper presented at Jackson Hole Rendezvous, Jackson Hole, WY.

Armstrong, S. (1997, March). *Compression viewed through multi-media glasses.* Paper presented at Seminars in Audition, Toronto, Ontario, Canada.

Armstrong, S. (1993). The dynamics of compression: Some key elements explored. *The Hearing Journal, 46*(11): 43–47.

Hickson, L. M. H. (1994). Compression amplification in hearing aids. *American Journal of Audiology, 3*(3): 51–65.

Johnson, W.A. (1993). Beyond AGC-O and AGC-I: Thoughts on a new default standard amplifier. *The Hearing Journal, 46*(11): 37–42.

Killion, M. C., Staab, W., & Preves, D. (1990). Classifying automatic signal processors. *Hearing Instruments, 41*(8): 24–26.

Killion, M. C. (1996). Compression; Distinctions. *The Hearing Review 3*(8): 29–32.

Killion, M. C. (1997). A critique on four popular statements about compression. *The Hearing Review, 4*(2): 36–56.

Kuk, F. (1999). Hearing aid design considerations for optimally fitting the youngest patients. *The Hearing Journal, 52*(4): 48–55.

Mueller, H. G., & Killion, M. C. (1996). Http://www.compression.edu. *The Hearing Journal, 49*(1): 10–46.

Staab, W. J., (December, 1996). Limiting systems in hearing aids. *AAS Bulletin, 21*(3): 23–31.

Venema, T. (2000). The many faces of compression. In R. E. Sandlin, (Ed.), *Handbook of hearing aid amplification* (2nd Ed). San Diego: Singular Publishing Group Inc.

6

Multi-Channel Programmable Hearing Aids

INTRODUCTION

In the last chapter we discussed the many types of compression, covering many of the "buzzwords" often encountered in the literature and in hearing aid specifications. A discussion of compression, however, would be incomplete without some discussion on multi-channel programmable hearing aids and how compression can be utilized in these types of circuits.

First, the terms "programmable" and "digital" should not be confused. Many high-end analog hearing aids of the late 1980s and mid 1990s were "digitally programmable," but this did not necessarily mean that the circuit of the hearing itself provided digital signal processing (DSP). The term "digitally programmable" simply meant that instead of requiring that the clinician employ a screwdriver, the hearing aid trimmer settings and/or VC could be programmed by a handheld programmer or by a computer with software created by some specific manufacturer. In summary, the only thing truly digital about these analog programmable hearing aids was the computer used to program them. Computers are truly digital because they process sound signals by the use a complex series of binary mathematical sequences (i.e., a series of 0's and 1's). The concept of "digital," along with the typical features of digital hearing aids, will be specifically covered in Chapter 7.

The high-end analog hearing aids of the mid 1990s were multi-channel hearing aids with WDRC in one or both channels. Many of these same hearing aids also had the added feature of being programmable. Today, almost all hearing aids are digital. What's more, almost all digital aids are multi-channel, and almost all digital hearing aids, are programmable. A proper understanding of this categorization demands clear definitions of the terms "multi-channel," and "programmable." This is the purpose of the present chapter.

The pace of hearing aid technology development that quickened in the early 1990s, continues at that same pace to this day. The major competition among hearing aid manufacturers also continues. Digital hearing aids that incorporate the use of multi-channels and programmability are being developed and released by the various hearing aid manufacturers at least as fast as this book is being written. This chapter, therefore, cannot intelligently cover an up-to-date competitive comparison and contrast of the features of multi-channel and programmability, as found in specific models of available hearing aids; rather the specific concepts of multi-channel and programmable are discussed here.

In the old days of the late 1980s to early 1990s, the first analog programmable hearing aids became available. These were all single-channel hearing aids. In the mid 1990s, analog nonprogrammable multi-channel hearing aids became available. Towards the late 1990s, most high-end analog hearing aids that were programmable also were multi-channel. The separate discussion of programmability and multi-channel begins here. Programmability will be discussed first, because it historically emerged first.

PROGRAMMABLE HEARING AIDS

The first programmable hearing aids were single-channel hearing aids where the clinician adjusted and set (i.e., programmed) the hearing aid trimmers with a computer or a handheld programming unit. Programmable hearing aids provide essentially the same compression characteristics as nonprogrammable hearing aids; the only difference is in the way that the controls or trimmers are accessed (programmability implies that no manual screwdriver manipulation is required). The only difference between programmable hearing aids and their nonprogrammable counterparts is that the clinician can set or adjust the trimmers by a computer or handheld programmer.

When programmable hearing aids first came out in the late 80s and early 90s, some four to eight different programs were often available for clinicians to set, and for clients to toggle among. It soon became evident that this number was far too cumbersome for the average client to deal with, so manufacturers began to drop the numbers of available programs to two or three.

Many programmable hearing aids thus offered two or three memories (i.e., programs); these programs provide clients access to different stored frequency responses with the flick of a switch, located on either the actual hearing aids, or on a hand-held remote-control device. By accessing different frequency responses, clients can personally adjust the hearing aids for optimal listening in different listening environments (Figure 6-1).

Some examples of programmable trimmer settings include: MPO, gain, low-cut, high-cut, compression threshold kneepoint, ratio of compression, and attack/release times. The software provided by various manufacturers might suggest some practical trimmer settings that tend to work well with each other, depending on the degree and slope of someone's hearing loss. The VC can also be programmed to be set at any particular position.

Programmable hearing aids can have one or more memories, or programs. Figure 6-2 shows an example of a two-program, single-channel hearing aid that is set to meet the needs of someone who wants the ability to choose between

Programmable versus Multi-Channel

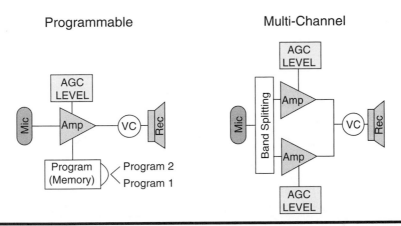

FIGURE 6–1 Programmable circuits can be single-channel or multi-channel. The programmable circuit (left) is a single-channel circuit with two memories or programs. This means the trimmer settings can be adjusted by either a handheld programmer or computer software. The listener can toggle between the two programs. One program might offer a more flat frequency response for listening in quiet, and the second program might offer less low-frequency gain and more high-frequency gain, which may be better for listening in background noise. The multi-channel circuit (right) could theoretically be available in either a programmable or a nonprogrammable format. Again, the trimmer settings can be adjusted by a handheld programmer or computer software. The multi-channel circuit shown above may have one or more memories or programs. If it has more than one program, the listener can adjust between or among different frequency responses for different listening situations. Most often, however, the properties of multi-channel and programmability are found together.

two different sound programs: one program that will provide optimal gain for listening in quiet or for listening to music, and so on, where the widest frequency response may be desired, and the other set for difficult listening situations, such as when trying to hear speech with background noise. For this person, the program for listening in quiet might be set to provide the necessary gain that comes closest to meeting the target(s) of a fitting method. The other program might be set to provide less low-frequency gain and more high-frequency gain, which could enable better or more comfortable listening in noise. This might result in a reduction of low-frequency background noise and more gain for the normally less intense, high-frequency consonants of speech. In summary, programmable hearing aids with more than one memory or program can be programmed to provide different clusters of trimmer settings for different listening situations.

There is more, however; different programmed memories can also provide alternate compression characteristics, or permit the client a choice between

An Example of Frequency Responses

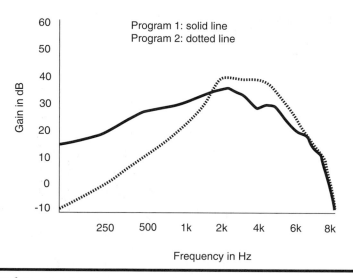

FIGURE 6–2   The frequency response for Program 1 of the fictitious programmable hearing aid shown here is adjusted to approach the target gain for soft speech inputs, established by some fitting method, for a fairly flat audiometric hearing loss. Program 2 is set to enable "better," perhaps more comfortable, listening to speech in noise. Program 1 has broader, flatter frequency response than Program 2. Program 2 provides more gain for the high frequencies and less gain for the low frequencies than Program 1. Theoretically, this should make the high-frequency consonants more audible to the listener and the low-frequency "hubbub" of background noise less audible. The listener can voluntarily toggle between the two programs, to best meet the need of each listening situation.

using directional versus omnidirectional microphone characteristics. For example, the programmed memories can each provide different microphone characteristics. One program can serve to provide omnidirectional sound, while another program provides directional sound. As will be discussed further in Chapter 8, directional microphones are not a new development in the hearing aid industry, but they currently are definitely receiving a lot of attention.

A big advantage of programmable hearing aids is that access to all parameters (e.g., low-cut, high-cut, gain, MPO, compression kneepoint, etc.) can be obtained through the computer or the handheld programmer. Not many ITEs can have a faceplate with more than three or four trimmers, because the "real estate," or space, on the faceplate cannot accommodate more than this number. If changes in nonprogrammable trimmers would be required, the clinician would need to return the hearing aid to the manufacturer. Programmability permits changes to any possible parameter or trimmer setting in the office, without the need to send the hearing aids back in to the manufacturer. A handheld programmer allows easy access and is especially convenient when programming the hearing aids at the client's residence.

Another advantage of programmability is that it enables more interaction between clinician and client. Both visual and auditory feedback are now available to clients when they can watch the programmed changes on the clinician's computer screen and at the same time can hear changes through the hearing aids. The visual input on the computer screen may also help to explain and illustrate the purpose and benefits of the hearing aids. Computers have gained acceptance in the public eye. Showing that hearing aid technology has kept in step with computer technology also prompts clients to accept their hearing aids more readily.

MULTICHANNEL HEARING AIDS

As we did for the discussion on programmability, the concept of multi-channel will be discussed in terms of how it was first implemented in the analog hearing aids of the mid 1990s. Multi-channel hearing aids are discussed here without relationship to programmability, and this is done for the purpose of clarity. Again, as mentioned earlier, multi-channel and programmability are two properties that are almost always found in combination, in the same hearing aid. This became the case for analog hearing aids, in the later 1990s. In fact, the high-end analog hearing aids at that time were explicitly known to be "programmable, multi-channel hearings aids with WDRC." In today's digital hearing aids, the properties of being programmable and multi-channel are almost always found together.

In 1995, the first analog multi-channel hearing aids with WDRC emerged. For the most part, analog multi-channel hearing aids had two channels, one representing the low frequencies and the other representing the high frequencies. ReSound introduced the first multi-channel products; others soon followed. One of the first two-channel hearing aids most familiar to the author was Unitron's Sound FX^{TM}. This product was built upon the popular Gennum DynamEQII^{TM} two-channel WDRC circuit. Only one analog multi-channel hearing aid had *three* channels, and that was the Clock^{TM} hearing aid produced by Argosy. With the advent of digital hearing aids, both of these products have long since disappeared from the marketplace.

Recall from Chapter 5 that all analog WDRC hearing aids also used input compression. This can be determined from the position of the VC, which is almost dead last in position in the two-channel circuit shown on the right side of Figure 6–1. Note that in the multi-channel hearing aid, there is one microphone, followed by a band splitter, which separates the incoming input sound into two frequency bands, or channels. Each frequency band or channel represents the low and high frequencies, respectively. Each separate channel has its own amplifier and compressor. On these high-end analog two-channel hearing aids, both BILL and TILL were commonly combined into one hearing aid, where BILL would be present in the low frequency channel and TILL would be present in

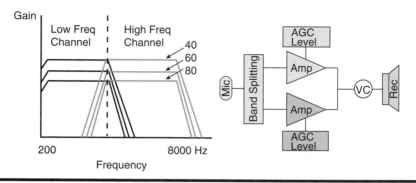

FIGURE 6–3   A two-channel WDRC hearing aid can be set up to produce a response of BILL, TILL, or both. If both channels have independent WDRC circuits, then the gain for both the low-frequency and high-frequency channels will increase for low-intensity input sound levels. On the right, a schematic for a two-channel compression hearing aid is shown. Following the microphone, a band splitter separates the inputs into a low-frequency band and a high-frequency band. Each frequency band is separately amplified and compressed. The end result is reunited into one receiver. There is also only one volume control. The gain and frequency graph on the left shows a two-channel WDRC hearing aid that is set up for both BILL and TILL. In this example, the client may have a "flat" hearing loss configuration.

the high-frequency channel (Figure 6–3). Since these high-end programmable, multi-channel hearing aids used WDRC, it could be assumed that they also used input compression.

The circuitry utilized in many of these high-end analog two-channel hearing aids allowed for a 12 dB/octave slope or a more steep 24 dB/octave slope between the two channels, as shown in Figure 6–4. When thinking about channels, the term "slope" refers to the steepness of the "sides" or "skirts" of the channels. The slope can be readily appreciated if the gain of one channel is turned down, while the gain of the other channel is turned way up. In Figure 6–4; the gain of the high-frequency channel rises dramatically above that provided by the low-frequency channel, at a rate of 24 dB/octave.

Compared to other analog hearing aids of the day, such a steep dB/octave slope between the two channels of these high-end analog hearing aids enhanced fitting flexibility. In analog hearing aid circuits, "passive" trimmers in hearing aids provided about a 6 dB/octave low-cut or high-cut effect on the frequency response of a hearing aid (Figure 6–4). "Active" low-cut or high-cut trimmers provided a more dramatic 12 dB to 18 dB/octave-effect. These also tended

Multi-Channel Hearing Aids Can Enable Steep Slope Between Channels

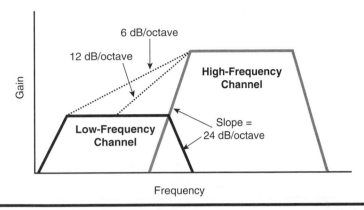

FIGURE 6–4   Analog "passive" low-cut or high-cut trimmers usually had a 6 dB/octave slope. "Active" trimmers had a 12 or 18 dB/octave slope, which enabled them to have more dramatic effects on the frequency response. A steep 24 dB/octave slope between two channels of a hearing aid enables independence between the channels, and consequently, even more flexibility in shaping the frequency response. It also helps to eliminate unwanted mid-frequency gain when this is desired (e.g., when fitting hearing losses that suddenly drop or improve). Two channels divided by a steep slope provide low- and high-frequency "plateaus," which can be raised or lowered with low-frequency and high-channel gain trimmers. In this example, the low-frequency channel gain is turned down while the high-frequency channel gain is turned up.

to cost more than passive trimmers. If the channels in a multi-channel hearing aid each had 6 dB or 12 dB/octave slopes, they would overlap considerably, and would not be very frequency-independent. The steep 24 dB/octave effect provided in the high-end analog two-channel hearing aids allowed even more independence between the two channels.

The advantage of such steep channel slopes became readily apparent to clinicians. The steep slopes enabled the ability to sculpt the gain/output of the hearing aid so that it could more closely fit difficult-to-fit audiometric configurations. The 24 dB/octave slope between the channels can eliminate unwanted mid-frequency gain when this is desired, for example, when fitting difficult-to-fit hearing losses that suddenly drop or improve. One example is the reverse or rising audiogram. Most people develop greater hearing loss for the mid to high frequencies; consequently, most hearing aids tend to provide greatest gain for the mid to high frequencies. Typical single-channel analog hearing aids of the day, often, provided too much mid- and high-frequency gain for the reverse hearing loss, even when using an active 12 dB/octave high-cut trimmer. Another example is the noise-induced hearing loss which tends to suddenly drop at around

F Control
Adjusting Where the Two Channels "Meet"

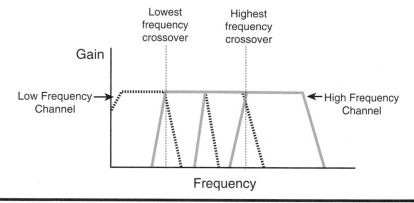

FIGURE 6–5   The frequency crossover control adjusts where the channels "meet." The whole purpose here is to increase fitting flexibility. The crossover control can be adjusted so the two channels meet anywhere from 500 Hz to about 2000 Hz. Its effects are completely independent from the gain controls for each channel. The "F" control can be thought of as the "horizontal" control, whereas the gain controls for each channel are the two "vertical" controls. Fitting flexibility with the high-end analog hearing aids of the mid to late 1990s was greatly enhanced for difficult-to-fit hearing loss configurations, such as reverse hearing losses and for precipitous high-frequency hearing losses.

2000 Hz. Again, the challenge with the typical hearing aids of the day for this challenging hearing loss was to provide sufficient gain for the high frequencies, without at the same time providing too much gain for the low and mid frequencies. Two channels divided by a steep slope provided low- and high-frequency "plateaus," which could be raised or lowered with the low- and high-channel gain trimmers. One could thus accommodate the "corner" in an audiogram, by providing very different amounts of gain for the low- versus the high frequencies.

In multi-channel hearing aids, the frequency region where the two channels "meet" can be adjusted by the crossover frequency control (Figure 6–5). Fitting flexibility is, thus, even further enhanced when the crossover frequency between the two channels can be adjusted. Accordingly, most two-channel analog hearing aids had an "F" control that adjusted the frequency crossover point where the channels came together. In general, the idea for clinicians is to adjust the frequency crossover control so that the two channels meet right at the frequency where the client's hearing changes the most. For example, if a hearing loss drops off suddenly at 2000 Hz, the crossover control can be adjusted so the two channels meet at 2000 Hz; the low- and high-frequency gain provided by

Gain for Each Channel Can Be Separately Adjusted
Increased Compression Ratio *Increases* Gain

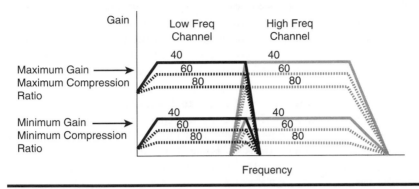

FIGURE 6–6   The overall gain for each channel is determined by the compression ratio selected for each channel. In many early multi-channel analog hearing aids, increased compression ratios resulted in increased gain. The purpose was to restore the normal growth of loudness for the client. Note here, however, that increased gain resulting from increased compression ratios does not change the relative amount of gain given to various input intensity levels. The distance among the gain line functions for maximum and minimum gain has not changed.

the low- and high-frequency channels could then be adjusted accordingly to provide the necessary (but different) amounts of gain for the low and high channels.

In the author's experience, probe microphone, or "real ear," measures of ear canal sound pressure levels typically revealed that the F control in these analog multi-channel hearing aids actually adjusted the frequency crossover from about 500 Hz to about 2000 Hz. When conducting seminars describing the "new" two-channel technology, the author recalls naming the low and high-frequency channel gain controls as "the vertical" controls, and the F control as the "horizontal" control.

The "vertical" controls (the gain of both channels) could independently be turned up or down. The low-frequency channel could be turned up while that of the high-frequency channel is turned down (Figure 6–6). This could be a good setting for a "reverse" hearing loss configuration. Conversely, the gain of the low channel could be turned down while that of the high channel was turned up. This could be a good setting for a high-frequency hearing loss. Lastly, if the gain of both channels was turned up the same, then the circuit provided a relatively flat amount of gain across the frequencies. With this advance in analog, multi-channel circuitry, it became easy for clinicians to see that one hearing aid circuit could serve clients with many varying degree of hearing loss, as well as many different hearing loss configurations. Fitting flexibility became the "name of the game." It is important for readers to know that this same gain flexibility in specific frequency channels is also available in today's digital hearing aids (Chapter 7).

Recall from Chapter 5 that both BILL and TILL are two types of WDRC, and that WDRC as a type of compression offers very different amounts of gain for soft versus intense input levels. Note from Figure 6–6, that the BILL or TILL per se, is not affected by the change in gain for the low- or high-frequency channels; only the overall gain is changed. This is evident in the fact that, when the gain for a channel is adjusted from minimum to maximum, the *difference* in gain for soft versus intense input levels does not change.

An especially interesting feature of many analog multi-channel hearing aid circuits (including the DynamEQII^{TM} circuit) was that the gain controls for the low- and high-frequency channels actually adjusted the *compression ratio* for each channel. This was indeed unusual, because up until this point in time, compression could only be adjusted by either an output limiting type of control or else, in the case of WDRC, a TK control. These types of controls adjust the "when" of compression, that is, the input level where compression would begin. The additional capability of adjusting the compression ratio enabled clinicians to adjust the amount or the "how much" of compression.

The way in which the gain was adjusted by compression ratio was also unique. In many of these high-end analog two-channel hearing aids, increased gain in the low- or high-frequency channels constituted an *increased* compression ratio (Figures 6–6, 6–7). In Chapter 5, we understood that compression is really a gain issue and that, compared to linear gain, compression provided less gain. That is, an input/output ratio of 2:1 normally provides less gain than an input/output ratio of 1:1. This understanding of compression is indeed true, provided that one assumes that on an input/output graph, the compression pivots from the left or lower kneepoint. The point here is that the compression ratio does not have to; it can also hinge from the right! If this is done, then linear (1:1) gain is less gain than, compression gain with, for example, a 2:1 ratio.

The input/output graph on the left side of Figure 6–7 is meant to represent any of the two channels of the analog, two-channel hearing aid discussed here. It shows that for each channel there are two kneepoints, a left or lower one and a right or higher one. Let's begin with the left-most or lower kneepoint, situated above the input SPL where compression "begins." As with all WDRC, the TK control adjusts the lower or left-most kneepoint. As discussed in Chapter 5, increasing the kneepoint with the TK control from 40 dB to 60 dB SPL inputs decreases the gain for soft input sounds, while decreasing the same kneepoint increases the gain for soft input sounds. This is because linear gain, provided below the kneepoint occurs for softer input levels.

Between the two kneepoints, the compression ratio on the multi-channel hearing aids typically ranged from 4:1 to 1:1. Recall from Chapter 5 that such ratios constitute WDRC. The unique thing in these hearing aids, unlike the other hearing aids of their day, was that the compression ratios "hinged" from the *right-most, higher* kneepoint, not from the first lower kneepoint. With this in mind, it becomes clear that as the compression ratio increases, so does the gain

Loudness Growth
&
Compression Ratios

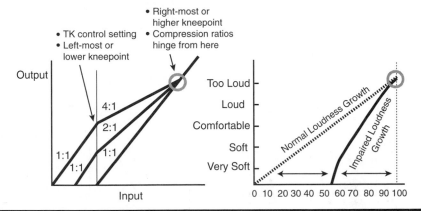

FIGURE 6–7 The relationship between loudness growth and compression ratios are shown here. In the right graph, the right arrow shows the dynamic range for someone's HL at some frequency; the left arrow shows required gain for various input levels required to restore normal loudness growth. The circle shows the "ceiling" of loudness tolerance for both SNHL and normal hearing. On the left is an input/output graph for one channel of a two-channel WDRC circuit, where the compression kneepoint as well as compression ratios can be adjusted. The circle again shows the output that corresponds to the "ceiling" of loudness tolerance on the right. The compression ratios hinge from this point. This higher kneepoint is fixed at some intensity corresponding to the circle shown in the right graph. The lines sloping to the left of the higher kneepoint show the adjustable ratios of compression needed to restore normal loudness growth. The diagonal lines rising from the X axis show the linear gain below the kneepoint of compression, which is adjusted by a TK control.

(Figure 6–7)! Again, this was quite contrary to most other types of compression, in which an increased compression ratio is associated with decreased gain.

The right-most or higher kneepoint is where compression "ends" (Figure 6–7). Beyond this input SPL, the hearing aid reached a point of "unity gain." Here, the compression ratio once again is linear, but there is no gain whatsoever. For example, a 95 dB input results in a 95 dB output, a 96 dB input results in a 96 dB output, and so on. Here, the hearing aid is truly acoustically "transparent."

The feature of adjusting compression ratios for the right-most or higher kneepoint was found to be very useful as a model for restoring normal loudness growth. The main idea behind this concept, first promoted by ReSound in the early 90s, was to restore normal loudness growth, as seen in Figure 6–7. The right side panel shows the reduced dynamic range and abnormal loudness growth that occurs with SNHL. It also shows the required gain to restore normal

TK Control at Lowest versus Highest Kneepoint Effects on Gain for Soft Inputs

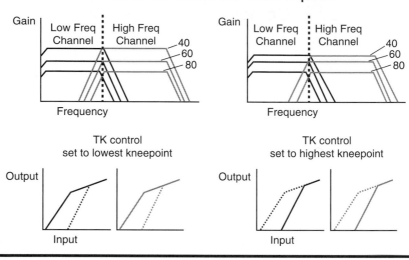

FIGURE 6–8   Note how the TK control adjustment does not affect the overall gain for all input intensity levels; on the contrary, it only affects the gain for soft inputs. The TK control changes the relative amount of gain given to various input intensity levels. As such, the distance among the gain line functions for maximum and minimum gain changes only for the 40 dB SPL input levels. Note also how the lower kneepoint set by the TK control increases the gain for soft inputs, and how a raised TK control setting decreases the gain for soft inputs.

loudness growth. The smaller dynamic range will require a greater amount of gain (greater compression ratio) to restore normal loudness growth. If the compression ratios hinge from an input level where one would want no gain at all, then soft sounds are given the most gain, while loud sounds are given little or no gain at all.

The feature of adjustable compression ratios separately for both channels was seen as a strong tool for restoring normal loudness growth. With increased compression ratio (increased gain), there is an approximation toward the ideal of restoring normal loudness growth. The TK control, at one time the only control available to adjust the compression of WDRC hearing aids, was now accompanied with adjustable compression ratios.

Adjustment of compression kneepoint and ratios should always be seen as two parts of a team (Figure 6–8). Compression ratios should be adjusted to best restore normal loudness growth for the client. To explain in the broadest terms, this means that for some frequency range, if the client's dynamic range is one half (about 50 dB) that of normal (about 100 dB), then adjust the compression ratio to 2:1. If the client's dynamic range is a quarter that of normal, then adjust the compression ratio so it is 4:1.

Recall from Chapter 5, that WDRC provides greatest (linear) gain for soft inputs below the kneepoint. The TK control at a lower position lowers the kneepoint of compression and increases the gain for soft input sounds. Setting the TK at the highest position raises the kneepoint as high as possible, but this reduces the overall effectiveness of the WDRC, which is to increase the gain for soft input sounds. The TK control would, therefore, theoretically always be set to the lowest kneepoint, so as to allow for the greatest possible amount of gain for soft input levels. Specifically, the TK control should be adjusted to provide as much gain for soft input sounds as possible, without at the same time resulting in feedback or the client's perception of a background "hiss." The TK control in these high-end analog hearing aids was, thus, basically used to address these complaints.

Look at the effects of the TK control adjustment versus low and high-channel gain adjustment (as seen in Figure 6–8). The multi-channel hearing aid is WDRC, as is evident with the very different amounts of gain provided for 40 dB versus 80 dB inputs. Note also, how the overall "height" of the gain lines is governed by the adjustment of the gain (or compression ratios) for each channel. The maximum gain for each channel, as we have seen already, is accomplished by maximum compression ratios for each channel (for example, 4:1). Compression ratio adjustment for each channel thus adjusts the amount of *overall gain* for each channel. Increasing the compression ratio raises the whole cluster of lines seen for the three input levels on Figure 6–8.

The TK control, on the other hand, determines the separateness or *distance* among the gain lines. Furthermore, it does so especially for the gains applied to 40 dB to 60 dB inputs, because the TK control adjusts the gain for soft inputs. The TK control, thus, adjusts the actual amount of BILL or TILL taking place within each channel. BILL is WDRC confined to the low frequencies, while TILL is WDRC confined to the high frequencies. The TK control thus adjusts the amount of WDRC in the hearing aid. In other words, it adjusts the amount of "spring" or "bounce" of the hearing aid; the difference in gain given to various input levels. This is after all, as we have seen in Chapter 5, why WDRC has been called "input level dependent compression." As types of WDRC, BILL and TILL have been referred to as, "frequency dependent compression."

We are now ready to look at digital hearing aids, how they incorporate compression and programmability across their various channels. As we shall see, digital hearing aids also offer lots more than this too.

SUMMARY

- This chapter basically serves to highlight the fact that the concepts of "programmability" versus "multi-channel" are separate concepts.
- Programmable hearing aids are discussed in conjunction with multi-channel hearing aids, because these two separate features were commonly found together in high-end analog hearing aids.
- The properties of having more than one channel and being programmable are shared by both analog and digital hearing aids.

- The terms "programmable" and "digital" should not be confused. For at least 10 years, from the late 1980s to late 1990s, many analog hearing aids were "digitally programmable"; as mentioned at the outset, the only digital about these hearing aids was the computer used to program them. This nomenclature only caused lots confusion on the part of consumers. Today, that whole point is moot, as almost all hearing aids are now digital.

REVIEW QUESTIONS

1. The term "programmable" means the hearing aid:
   a. has two or more channels.
   b. has two or more programs.
   c. is digital.
   d. settings can be adjusted by software instead of by a screwdriver.

2. Multi-channel" means that:
   a. clients can switch among different frequency responses.
   b. clients can switch among different channels.
   c. the hearing aid is programmable.
   d. the hearing has more than one frequency band or channel.

3. The term "digitally programmable" means the hearing aid is:
   a. digital.
   b. analog.
   c. multi-channel.
   d. none of the above

4. The following statement is false:
   a. Programmable hearing aids can be single or multi-channel.
   b. Multi-channel hearing aids can be programmable or nonprogrammable.
   c. Nonprogrammable hearing aids cannot be multi-channel.
   d. Programmable hearing aids can have a single memory (program).

5. The following statement is true:
   a. "Programmable" means the hearing aid has more than one channel.
   b. Hearing aids can be multi-channel and programmable with more than one program.
   c. "Multi-channel" means clients can switch between different frequency responses.
   d. Hearing aids cannot be multi-channel and programmable with more than one program.

6. In programmable hearing aids, a typical number of programs or memories is:

    a. one.

    b. two or three.

    c. four or five.

    d. six or seven.

7. A typical number of channels for the high-end analog multi-channel hearing aids of the last decade was:

    a. one.

    b. two.

    c. three.

    d. four.

8. Active band or channel slopes are typically at least:

    a. 6 dB/octave.

    b. 12 dB/octave.

    c. 24 dB/octave.

    d. 48 dB/octave.

9. For compression that hinges from a right-most kneepoint:

    a. linear gain is the least gain.

    b. linear gain is the most gain.

    c. more compression means more gain.

    d. more compression means less gain.

10. The DynamEQII^{TM} circuit from Gennum was:

    a. a single-channel, analog circuit that provided two programmable memories.

    b. a single-channel, single-program analog hearing aid with both BILL and TILL.

    c. a linear hearing aid circuit of the 1980s.

    d. none of the above

RECOMMENDED READINGS

Staab, W. J. (1990). Digital/programmable hearing aids—An eye toward the future. *British Journal of Audiology, 24,* 243–256.

Venema, T. H. (2000). The many faces of compression. In R. Sandlin (Ed.), *Hearing aid amplification* (pp. 1–35). Singular, Thomson Delmar, Inc.

7

Digital Hearing Aids

INTRODUCTION

So far, the reader no doubt wonders why it has taken up until this point to finally and specifically address digital hearing aids. True, we have consistently referred to digital hearing aids as something to be discussed later on. But it is the author's strong opinion that digital hearing aids cannot be truly appreciated unless the characteristics of their analog forebears are understood. As mentioned earlier in Chapter 5, compression in analog hearing aids had to be understood because those hearing aids typically provided either one type or another type of compression. Successful client fittings relied on such knowledge. That is why decade of the 1990s was truly the golden age of compression. Furthermore, programmability and the property of multi-channel amplification (as discussed in Chapter 6) also originated in analog hearing aids.

These advances in amplification are now "de rigour" in today's digital hearing aids. Digital hearing aids are almost all adjusted by the manufacturer's fitting software. The gain, MPO, compression, and much more, are adjusted and implemented by means of software, on to the hardware of the digital chip, or, the digital signal processing (DSP) core. Compression characteristics and all kinds of other features are automatically combined and separately adjusted on each frequency band or channel of the digital hearing aid, at the flick of the software's "quick-fit" option. As mentioned in Chapter 5, the one drawback of this (in the author's opinion) is that so much seems buried this way. Clinicians who do not take the time to understand the rationales behind the software's settings are in peril of becoming mere technicians who just push buttons and who don't understand "why." Here, it is important for clinicians to determine which digital hearing aids they most often recommend, and then to actually *listen* to these hearing aids in various environments. Compare the sound quality of different digital hearing aids when they are set up to meet the fitting requirements of some specific hearing loss. Do not completely rely on the marketing claims made by the manufacturers; take the time to check them out with your own

Analog and Digital Hearing Aid Circuits

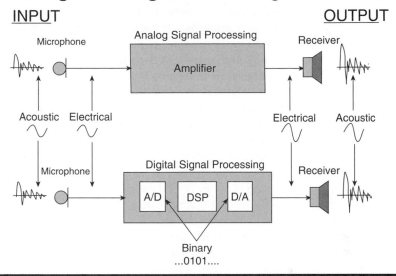

INPUT   OUTPUT

FIGURE 7–1   All hearing aid circuits (analog and digital) have a microphone and a receiver. The difference between the analog and the digital circuit is the processing that takes place between the microphone and the amplifier. In the analog circuit, there is a change from sound into electricity at the microphone; from there, the amplifier adds gain and at the receiver, the sum total is changed back into sound. In the digital circuit, the microphone also changes sound into electricity but then, the analog-to-digital (A/D) converter changes the electricity into numbers. Here the gain is added (along with other elements of DSP). Past this point, the digital-to-analog (D/A) converter changes the numbers back into electricity. From there, the receiver changes the electricity back into sound.

ears. Recall from Chapter 5 and its discussion on compression types; the cochlea is an excellent acoustic analyzer.

"Digital" versus "Analog"

All hearing aids that do not have a digital circuit, or a DSP core, are analog hearing aids. For hearing aids, the term "analog" means that the patterns of electrical current or voltages in the circuit are analogous (similar) to those of the acoustic (sound) input. It is also important to remember the electrical patterns are continuous (not discrete pieces), just like the incoming and outgoing sound waves. When thinking of analog, think about sound being played from old-time record albums on a stereo turntable. The needle wiggles in the grooves on the record, and these wiggle patterns are converted into analogous patterns of electricity, which are then amplified. These amplified patterns of electricity are then turned back into sound waves by the speakers (which are like microphones in reverse). Figure 7–1 shows a very simple schematic of an analog hearing aid circuit compared to that of a digital hearing aid circuit. Note that the analog circuit includes two different kinds of energy: acoustic (i.e., sound) and electrical (i.e., voltage and current).

Both analog and digital hearing aids share the fact that they all have microphones and receivers, known as *transducers*. Transducers simply change energy from one form into another (microphones change sound into electricity and the receiver changes electricity back into sound). At the amplifier stage, gain is added to the input, and the sum total electrical current or voltage is sent on to the receiver, where it is converted back into sound. Transducers like microphones and receivers, for the most part, are all analog.

As Figure 7-1 shows, digital hearing aids have an *additional* transduction process; after the sound is transduced into electricity by the microphone, an analog-to-digital (A/D) converter changes the electrical current into binary sequences of numbers (or digits). These digits can be manipulated in almost any way possible to provide the gain or other digital processing instructions that are needed for someone's hearing requirements. Once the DSP algorithms have been executed (i.e., once the binary digits have been manipulated), the numbers are then changed back into electrical current by a digital-to-analog (D/A) converter. This current is then transduced back into sound by the receiver.

When reading about digital hearing aids, one may encounter the term "algorithm," which is simply a series of mathematical instructions. Numbers lend themselves easily to manipulation, and this ability is what makes digital hearing aids very attractive. Digital circuitry allows the frequency response of the hearing aid to be even more flexible than that of the analog, multi-channel WDRC hearing aids (described in Chapter 6). With DSP, the frequency response can be literally "sculpted" to meet the target(s) of gain as closely as possible. Additional digital algorithms provide other, unparalleled flexibility and adaptability not easily accomplished with analog circuitry. More advantages of digital hearing aids are described later.

The basic thing to remember about digital hearing aids is that sound is represented and manipulated by separate or discrete (not continuous) numbers or digits. When reading about digital hearing aids, various terms are encountered: two of these are "sampling rate" and "quantization." These refer to the way a digital circuit converts a continuous analog signal into a sequence of discrete numbers. In more simple terms, these terms refer to the way in which the frequency and the intensity of sound become represented by numbers. Figure 7-2 shows the basic concepts behind sampling rate and quantization. The sampling rate is how often the digital circuit samples the amplitude of the analog signal, per some unit of time. In other words, the sampling rate is the frequency of sampling (seen as the horizontal axis of Figure 7-2). If the sampling rate is fast, these times between the samples taken is very small. A digital circuit with a fast sampling rate "samples" the sound more often as the sound changes over time than does a digital circuit with a slower sampling rate. The higher the sampling rate, the greater the ability for the digital circuit to accurately represent very high frequencies of sound with numbers. High frequencies have very short periods, or cycle times for each wavelength to occur. To represent these short wavelengths

Sampling & Quantization

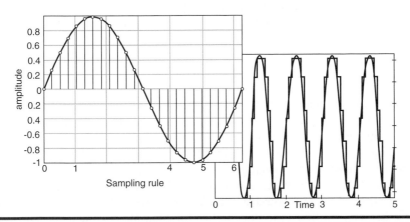

FIGURE 7–2   The graph on the left shows the incoming sound wave and how it becomes represented by numbers (digits) in a DSP hearing aid. A sound wave always shows amplitude on the vertical axis, and time along the horizontal axis. Sampling rate of the DSP circuit is the frequency that the sound is represented with numbers (digits), and these are shown on the horizontal axis. The vertical lines on the left-most graph show the sound as it is sampled over time. If these lines were closer together, the sampling rate would be faster. Quantization of the DSP circuit represents intensity with numbers (digits), and these are shown on the vertical axis. The graph on the right shows the sound wave (on the left) as it is represented digitally.

accurately with numbers requires a fast sampling rate that represents the sound over very small units of time.

Quantization is the ability of the DSP circuit to accurately represent the sound intensity (Figure 7–2, vertical axis). Quantization is the assignment of numbers to the samples of sound, where the numbers represent voltages or current levels. Quantization thus generates a stream or series of numbers that represent the sampled signal level. As with the sampling rate, more quantization permits more accuracy of intensity representation by numbers. A sound wave that can be assigned, for example, 65,536 possible intensity values is far more accurately represented than the same sound wave when assigned, say, 256 possible intensity values. In the former case, each of many different specific intensities can be assigned a specific numerical value. In the latter case, intensities that are located between any one of the 256 possible values will have to be rounded up or down to the closest value. A high amount of quantization, thus, enables low distortion and a high dynamic range; in other words, very soft sounds as well as loud sounds can be captured or represented digitally. A high sampling rate together with many possible quantized values is like a fine-toothed comb: It permits a higher resolution or a more accurate numeric representation of the sound. Obviously, a high degree of quantization and a high sampling rate are preferred, but these may come with a cost—namely, high-power consumption. A complete discussion of digital hearing aids is beyond the scope of this book (and the author's knowledge); however, some specific digital advances are roughly sketched in this chapter, along with some of the main ways in which digital hearing aids use compression.

Open Platform versus Closed Platform

At the initial advent of digital hearing aids (late 1990s), electrical engineers at various manufacturers often discussed the terms "open platform" and "closed platform." These refer to the degree to which the digital hearing aids could be software driven. A truly *open platform* digital product would be similar to a regular computer; it would have hardware that would be able to run all kinds of software, from word processing to hearing aid compression characteristics. This would enable complete freedom to provide whatever it takes to meet the needs of your client (Pavlovic, Bisgaard, & Melanson, 1998). But then, too much freedom is not necessarily a good thing either; for example, no one truly wants to do word processing with a hearing aid either. Again, this would require far too much processing power and consequent battery drain.

In view of hearing aid fittings, open platform DSP would enable complete flexibility, so that, on any one hearing aid, totally different characteristics can be downloaded by software. On a single open platform digital hearing aid, a continuum of completely different hearing aids could be created by software, from a linear, single-channel hearing aid to a two-channel WDRC hearing aid, to a 10-channel hearing aid where each channel had its own specific parameters of input compression WDRC and output limiting compression. All parameters such as filters, directionality, MPO, and so on can be written in software (Edmonds, Staab, Preves, & Yanz, 1998). The main disadvantage of a completely open platform digital hearing aid is that, at this time, it would have to be quite large and it would draw a lot of battery power; besides, the final end-product software might not be so very different from that used in closed platform digital hearing aids (Kuk, 1998).

Another disadvantage that comes to mind is the fact that clinicians might not know what to do with all the flexibility offered by a truly open platform digital hearing aid. In fact, this is why "quick fit" options appear on today's fitting software; so many possible software adjustments are available on some products, that well-meaning clinicians simply are overwhelmed by them.

A *closed platform* digital product has constraints built into the hardware that make the hearing aid dedicated to specific digital functions, such as having channels that represent bands of frequency. The digital functions inside the closed platform digital hearing aid cannot be changed at will, because the hearing aid hardware itself is dedicated to performing certain functions. According to Kuk (1998), a closed platform DSP hearing aid is similar to an open platform DSP hearing aid, except that the manufacturer has elected to include in the hardware only portions necessary to provide benefit to the end user. As mentioned earlier, an advantage of closed platform is that the power consumption and size can be kept to a minimum. All of today's digital hearing aids are essentially closed platform; it's just that some are more closed than others.

One main advantage of DSP is that various compression schemes or combinations can be incorporated numerically, without many of the constraints of analog circuits. Digital hearing aids also offer the following list of advantages over their analog counterparts, and these are each discussed below, in this chapter

1. In situ audiometric testing
2. Many more than two or three channels
3. Automatic feedback reduction
4. Combined types of compression in each channel
5. Expansion (the opposite of compression for very soft inputs)
6. Digital noise reduction (DNR) or speech enhancement features

IN SITU TESTING

One thing not commonly mentioned about digital hearing aids is the fact that they can sometimes produce as well as receive sounds! For example, *in situ* behavioral thresholds can be measured; this means a behavioral audiogram can be produced with the hearing aid in place in the client's ear canal (Ludvigsen & Topholm, 1997). The hearing aid gain and output can then be adjusted to best meet target as specified by some fitting method. Such direct measures like these overcome the necessity to manually transfer data back and forth from the audiogram in dB HL to the hearing aid in dB SPL. Even more importantly, direct in-situ measures reduce the errors that commonly appear with transforms from behavioral thresholds obtained under headphones, to 2 cc coupler data, to probe tube real-ear measures. In other words, in situ thresholds can remove the seams from the hearing aid fitting process. Digital hearing aids that can produce sounds are also capable of self diagnostic testing (Auriemo, Nielson, & Kuk, 2003).

DIGITAL ARCHITECTURE: CHANNELS AND BANDS

Whereas high-end analog hearing aids are almost always restricted to two frequency bands or channels, digital hearing aids are known to have in excess of 20 bands or channels! Here is a good point to distinguish between "bands" and "channels."

In analog hearing aids, the term "frequency band" was used interchangeably with the term "channel." These bands or channels were often separated by filtering, from other frequency regions. In Chapter 6, and in Figure 6-1, this filtering was referred to as "band splitting." In each band, only the gain—and consequently, the output—was adjusted. For today's digital hearing aids, much more than gain can be adjusted independently in each frequency band. It has become industry convention to posit that if only the gain is adjusted, each frequency region is called a "band." This is just convention; there is no official definition of "bands" and "channels." So, if the whole point is shaping the frequency response, then one might call such a hearing aid a "multi-band" system.

On the other hand, if more than just the gain is adjusted within a band, then the band would be referred to as a "channel." Lots more than just gain can be adjusted within a band, for example, specific types of compression, such as BILL or TILL, or noise reduction, or feedback reduction. In today's digital hearing aids, therefore, channels are groups of frequency bands that share a digital algorithm. For example, if a group of low-frequency bands has a digital algorithm that instructs it to provide BILL, this group would comprise a low-frequency BILL channel. In the final analysis, it is possible to have more bands than channels, but not the other way around. From now one, let's just use the term "channel."

The dB/octave slope of the individual channels in digital hearing aids can be much steeper than in analog hearing aids, and this further increases fitting flexibility. The steepest analog slope found in hearing aids is 24 dB/octave. An example was Gennum's DynamEQ™ circuit, as mentioned in Chapter 6. Although a 24 dB/octave slope permits a relative degree of independence between channels, it does not allow complete independence. With DSP, the slope between adjacent channels can be almost infinitely steep compared to those of analog multi-channel hearing aids. A very steep slope between channels permits an even higher degree of fitting flexibility for various shapes or configurations of hearing loss than that already obtained with analog multi-channel WDRC hearing aids. By adjusting the gain and output of each channel, much like the buttons on a stereo equalizer, the frequency response can be literally "sculpted" to meet the target (or targets) of gain as closely as possible (Figure 7–3).

At this point, it is very important to mention a digital hearing aid that has been available for the past few years; namely, the Symbio™ produced by Bernafon. This product is presently marketed to clinicians as being "channel-free." Many have asked what this means. Specifically, what is the difference between having one channel and being channel-free? Technical explanations for the difference abound, but few understand them. At the risk of stumbling into a quagmire of jargon, an attempt will be made here to sketch out a palatable explanation of the concept of "channel-free." The specific purpose of this little discussion is to highlight the various types of DSP *architecture* that can be found in today's digital hearing aids.

In the beginning of the digital hearing aid era (1996–1997), digital hearing aids were construed and developed as digital versions of their analog counterparts. In Chapter 6, we looked at programmable, multi-channel hearing aids as they appeared in their analog form. When digital hearing aids first emerged, their architecture was constructed so as to digitally imitate the analog properties that came before them. Recall that in analog multi-channel hearing aids, the microphone sent the input to a band-splitter (filter), which separated the input into frequency-specific bands. Thus, the typical analog multi-channel hearing aid had a low- and a high-frequency band, and each band was separately adjustable in terms of gain. After being separately processed, the final results in each channel were then recombined together. This end-product was sent out to the receiver, which transduced the electrical product into an acoustic product for

Increased Number of Lots of Frequency Bands
Increases Accurate Hz Shaping / Fitting Flexibility

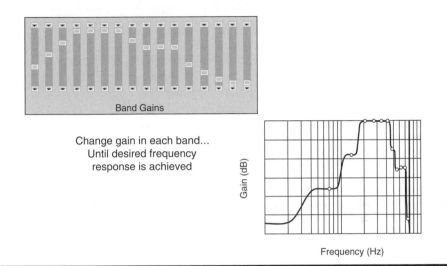

Band Gains

Change gain in each band...
Until desired frequency
response is achieved

Gain (dB)

Frequency (Hz)

FIGURE 7–3   A fictitious frequency band equalizer is shown in the left panel. Each button represents a particular frequency channel. Selective adjustment of adjacent buttons would allow an exquisite sculpting of the frequency response, as shown in the right panel. Digital hearing aids are mostly multi-channel. Their dB/octave slopes can be almost infinite, meaning that adjacent frequency bands can be very independent from each other. Turning the gain up on one band may thus not affect the gain in adjacent bands.

"consumption" by the human ear. Concepts like this were understood by clinicians, so when digital technology began in the hearing aid manufacturing sector, it was far easier to re-create them in digital form, and then add to them as technology advanced.

Most electrical engineers admit that in digital hearing aids, splitting input sound into separate, parallel bands or channels, processing the sound in each individual band or channel, and then reuniting them back together, is not always such a good idea, because it invites unwanted distortion. Today, this unwanted distortion has largely been dealt with and overcome (S. Armstrong, 2005, personal communication).

In hindsight, however, an electrical engineer purist would not have taken things this route. But many hearing aid manufacturers did. They did so because of natural hearing aid evolution. It was the custom, so it was correct. This, in and of itself, is testimony to what was said at the outset of Chapter 5; namely, *it is very important for aspiring clinicians to understand the advances made in analog hearing aids before digital technology can truly be appreciated!*

Since most digital hearing aids divide the frequency response into bands or channels, perhaps we should discuss how this can be achieved. There are

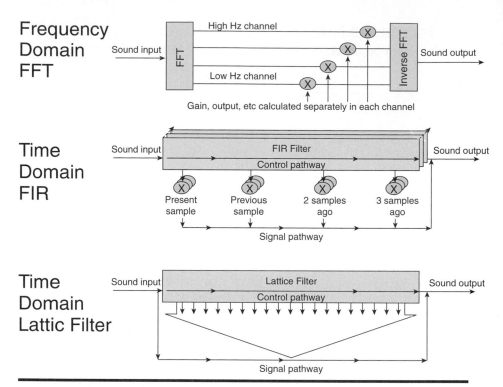

FIGURE 7–4 Digital hearing aids present with various forms of architecture. The top panel shows digital signal processing (DSP) in the frequency domain, accomplished by means of a fast Fourier transform (FFT). This results in a simultaneous parallel processing of narrow bands of frequency bands in separate channels. The middle panel shows DSP in the time domain as it occurs with cascaded finite impulse response (FIR) filters. These are shown as the three long rectangle boxes superimposed on each other. Note that the control path is constantly fed into the signal path, resulting in a continuous serial processing of sound inputs over tiny units of time. The usage of cascaded FIR filters still results in fixed frequency channels. The bottom panel also shows DSP in the time domain; the difference here is that the processing is accomplished by means of a lattice filter, where the breakage of sound inputs into separate channels is not evident.

various available forms of DSP architecture for hearing aids; some operate in the *frequency* domain, and some in the *time* domain (Figure 7-4). Because the first digital hearing aids divided the frequency response into a small number channels, they could operate in the time domain. When this is the case, a finite impulse response (FIR) is part of the digital signal processing (DSP) architecture (Armstrong, 2005, personal communication). This is the simplest method of digitally producing a frequency response filter. For a small number of channels, an FIR filter is clearly the most efficient.

Many digital hearing aids today operate in the time domain using an FIR filter. An FIR filter assigns any one of a finite series of many quantization values to each successive sample of the input over time. If, for example, there is a finite number of 20,000 samples taken per second, a new sample can be quantized every 50 micro seconds. Think about this: A millisecond is one thousandth of a second; a microsecond is one millionth of a second. First, the desired output frequency response—based on the hearing loss, the fitting method used, and any other selected option provided by the fitting software—is fed into the hearing aid. The FIR filter then assigns some quantized value to each new input sample taken, in accordance with specific output demands that are placed upon it, so as to achieve the desired output frequency response. Each new sample thus quantized, is added to *all the other samples* that have previously quantized, in order to constantly update the *entire* output frequency response over time. One can think of the FIR filter as an equalizer operating over time, where the buttons adjust sound along three dimensions (e.g., amplitude, frequency, and sharpness).

In the construction of digital hearing aids, several FIR filters aligned together create fixed channels (T. Scheller, 2005, personal communication; L. Cornelisse, 2005, personal communication). For channels situated between the lowest and highest frequency channels, two FIR filters are required to produce one channel, one for the low-frequency side and another for the high-frequency side of the channel. The lowest-frequency channel would only have a high-frequency FIR filter, and the highest-frequency channel would only have a low-frequency FIR filter. Thus, an eight-channel digital hearing aid operating in the time domain with FIR filters would present with some 14 FIR filters. Earlier examples of such systems operating in the time domain using FIR filters were the Senso™ from Widex, and the DigiFocus™ from Oticon. More will be discussed on these two pioneering digital hearing aids later on in this chapter (under the section, "Two Examples of Early Digital Hearing Aids"). Today, the Foundation™ and the Paragon™ are examples of time domain digital platforms, which are produced by Gennum; these are incorporated in two low-end digital hearing aids from Unitron.

As the number of channels increased, a different method of dividing the frequency range becomes more efficient (Figure 7–4). This method operates in the frequency domain, employing a fast Fourier transform (FFT). The FFT acts as a digital filter to split the incoming sound, analyses its frequency content and split the incoming signal into separate parallel frequency bands. The gain, compression, etc., in each of these bands are then separately manipulated according to the digital algorithms of the hearing aid. Once this is done, the separate contents of each parallel frequency band are reunited and sent on out to the receiver to be transduced back into acoustic form. Adjustment of separate individual channels in these FFT systems is similar to that of the typical equalizer, with buttons that represent only frequency.

At this point, it may be useful to discuss the issue of *processing time delay*, something that occurs in all hearing aids. This time delay is measured in the order of milliseconds. Any frequency response filtering necessarily requires processing time, even in analog circuits. Digital systems, however, always take more time to accomplish the same filtering than do analog systems. Such time delays (sometimes referred to as "group delays") range from several to 10 or more milliseconds. One can begin to actually hear the time delay when it approaches 20 milliseconds. With longer processing time delays, if you clapped your hands while listening to the hearing aid, you would hear a small delay in the aided clap. Since most digital hearing aids today have shorter processing times (including those with FFT systems operating in the frequency domain), this audible "echo" is not often a problem. Still, however, processing times that create even short time delays threaten to create *distorted sound quality*. For a very interesting read on processing time delay in digital products, the reader is encouraged to look at a past American Academy of Audiology presentation, given by Henrickson in 2004.

It may be good to summarize a few rather interesting points regarding time delay in the frequency domain versus the time domain. Digital hearing aids with FFT systems operating in the frequency domain tend to require more time delay than their cousins operating in the time domain. For these digital hearing aids, time must enter the picture because any signal processing necessarily requires some time to occur. The more filters (or channel divisions) these hearing aids have, the more processing time is required. Frequency domain digital hearing aids incorporate the use of small "windows" of time, where all the samples from each parallel frequency band within each successive window are processed as a unit (Schmidt, 2005, personal communication). These digitally processed windows of digitally sampled information are successively moved along to the receiver, like small packages along an incredibly fast conveyor belt, from the DSP core to the receiver. The length of time delay in these hearing aids is equal to the length of the processing windows.

For digital hearing aids operating in the frequency domain, more, narrower channels require longer time windows and thus, longer time delays. An advantage here, however, is that higher "order" filters are more readily available than in those digital hearing aids operating in the time domain (Schmidt, 2005, personal communication). In other words, the slopes of the channel sides (as discussed previously in Chapter 6) can be made to be extremely steep, without requiring much more processing power. When more than 12 dB/octave roll-off is provided for the channel slopes, crossover between adjacent frequency bands is minimized. Adjacent frequency bands in these digital hearing aids often sit side-by-side like two walls, enabling incredible frequency shaping. The processing time delay, however, necessarily increases with increased number of narrow frequency channels. Digital processing in the frequency domain, with lots of steeply sloped frequency channels, can thus result in degraded sound quality. Obviously, the developers of these types of DSP systems realize this and have taken means to reduce the distortion. This does not come without a cost; such distortion reduction requires additional processing power.

Digital hearing aids operating in the time domain generally tend to require more processing power than those operating in the frequency domain. An advantage for digital hearing aids operating in the time domain, however, is that they present with comparatively very little processing time delay. Another thing to note here is that for digital hearing aids that use FIR filters, the *steep slopes* of the channel "walls" imply more time delay, not the greater number of channels per se.

There are other possible types of digital filters that could be used, but these two (FIR and FFT) are most often currently employed in today's commercially available digital hearing aids. All of these digital hearing aids operating in the time domain with FIR filters, and in the frequency domain using FFTs, have *fixed* channels. There are other possible permutations or combinations of FFTs and FIR filters, and these are also utilized in today's digital hearing aids. The recent Innova™ from Sonic Innovations is an example of this. The Symbio™ by Bernafon, however, stands out as quite unique, among all of these.

"Channel-free" digital processing is the direction taken by the developers of the Symbio™. This digital hearing aid does indeed operate in the time domain. Instead of using FIR filters, however, as these other hearing aids do, the Symbio™ uses something called a "lattice" filter (Figure 7–4). Like other time domain systems using FIR filters, lattice filtering enables frequency response shaping by updating the frequency response *very rapidly* over tiny, *serial* units of time. It is quite adjustable, and alters the input sound in terms of its frequency response and its input/output characteristics. That is, the lattice filter defines the appropriate frequency response, based on the hearing loss of the client, as according to the clinician's fitting method, etc.

Unlike the other time domain systems using FIR filters (or the frequency domain systems using FFTs, for that matter), however, the lattice filter does not result in fixed channels (Scheller, 2005, personal communication). Recall our earlier discussion on time domain digital processing systems, where we noted that channel divisions were still evident in digital hearing aids that utilize FIR filters; the use of the lattice filter in the Symbio™ seems to enable a "holistic" sculpting of the output frequency response without an apparent channel division. Just how this is accomplished, however, is entirely beyond the electrical engineering knowledge base of the author. The end-result (the required output frequency response) is achieved, but the method of getting there is very different from that offered by other digital hearing aids.

It should be noted that the Symbio™ does not provide digital noise reduction as a feature, like many other digital hearing aids do. Fixed, separate frequency bands, as found in many other digital hearing aids are quite useful for implementing such features as noise reduction (more will be discussed on the noise reduction feature later on in this chapter). In order to provide digital noise reduction, the Symbio™ would have to add noise reduction as a completely separate feature or system, independently of its "channel-free" processing. This would undoubtedly and substantially increase its time delay, which would, in turn, compromise its sound quality. For a product where the initiative is to maximize sound quality, this would not be a sought-after feature. Still, however, many experienced hearing aid wearers subjectively comment that the Symbio™ has unusually good overall sound quality.

In summary, there are always trade-offs to be considered when engineering new digital hearing aids. It behooves of clinicians to *listen to digital products with their own ears*, and compare sound quality among digital hearing aids before automatically adhering to the claims of the manufacturers who build them. The cochlea is a wonderfully accurate analyzer of sound. The high-end digital hearing aid from any one specific manufacturer may not necessarily offer the best sound quality. Sometimes, the simpler products, with fewer frequency bands and fewer bells and whistles in fact sound the best!

AUTOMATIC FEEDBACK REDUCTION

Automatic feedback reduction is another digital feature. Feedback is one of the major complaints of hearing aid wearers. It is caused when aided sound outputs from the receiver leak out of the ear canal, either through a slit leak because the hearing aid is loosely fit or through a vent. These outputs can then be picked up by the microphone and passed through the hearing aid again. This sound loop then becomes repetitive until the cycle is somehow stopped, either by reducing the gain or the input. Feedback most often can occur when a hand or telephone is placed close to the aided ear; any sound leaking from the receiver back to the microphone is thus actually enhanced, because it is literally guided to the microphone by bouncing off the hand or the telephone receiver. Feedback is noted by large, sharp peaks in the mid- to high-frequency response of the hearing aid output (Figure 7–5). Besides being annoying, feedback can also drive an amplification system into its MPO, and thereby reduce battery life (Chabries & Bray, 2002).

Feedback reduction is generally accomplished by reducing the narrow, sharp peaks that appear in the hearing aid's output frequency response. In many digital hearing aids, feedback that does occur can be automatically sensed and reduced. Automatic feedback reduction can also reduce the need for filters, which tend to easily clog up with wax.

Hayes (2003) writes a concise article that reviews some of the techniques and challenges in reducing feedback in digital hearing aids today. The usual approaches to feedback reduction are the use of notch filters or phase canceling. Notch filters simply reduce the gain in a narrow frequency range and, thus, can reduce the sharp feedback peaks in the output frequency response. If the feedback peaks would always occur at the same narrow band of frequencies, then a static notch filter set to reduce the gain at the same narrow band of frequencies would work very well. Furthermore, according to Hayes (2003), this approach would create very little increase in battery consumption and digital processing demands. The trouble is that most feedback peaks are not always so stable; changes in the listening environment create changes in the locations of feedback peaks.

"Roving" notch filters address this problem to some degree, but they also consume more battery and digital processing power (Hayes, 2003). These roving

Automatic Feedback Reduction
Reduces the need for filters

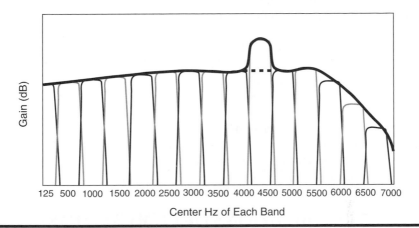

FIGURE 7–5 Feedback is caused by mid- to high-frequency peaks in a frequency response. Reduction of such peaks eliminates the feedback. In digital hearing aids, these peaks can be reduced mathematically without the need for physical filters. In analog hearing aids, filters were used to reduce peaks that could potentially cause feedback. These filters, however, could easily clog up, due to wax, perspiration, etc. All too often, the presence of a clogged filter meant a functionless hearing aid.

notch filters tend to be limited to reducing a maximum of three feedback peaks, because the usage of more such notch filters can compromise the frequency response. Lastly, the roving notch filters set to operate on some three peaks will require some time (some 200 milliseconds) to lock on to the offending feedback peaks.

Another approach to feedback is phase cancellation. The feedback peak (or peaks) are detected, and then reverted into opposite phase. This opposite phase signal is then used to cancel out the feedback. The phase canceling itself is done at the microphone stage of the feedback (Hayes, 2003). Phase canceling is a potentially powerful tool to suppress feedback peaks: like the roving notch filter approach, however, phase canceling often can require increased battery and digital signal processing power. Phase canceling also faces the challenges posed by the necessity of tracking feedback peaks that are constantly changing. The time required to accurately track and revert phase to changing feedback peaks can be a half a second.

A different and less computationally demanding technique to reduce feedback is utilized by Unitron Hearing, namely, the Real Time Feedback Canceller™ (Hayes, 2003). This approach detects feedback peaks separately in each narrow frequency band, instead of using a single model of the feedback signal path with all of its frequencies together. As such, it places less demands on battery consumption and digital signal processing. It also reacts in less than 100 milliseconds, which is far quicker than the phase cancellation approach.

According to Walesa (2005, personal communication), the Real Time Feedback Canceller™ sits somewhere in between the notch filter and the phase cancellation approaches. Its focus is to reduce feedback early on, as they occur in each frequency band of the digital hearing aid. It detects small feedback peaks before they can grow larger. In short, it can be seen as the prevention instead of the cure, or, as Walesa (2005) posits, "like ABS brakes instead of air bags." It is especially effective at quickly reducing feedback resulting from reflective surfaces; it cannot claim, however, to maximize available gain as the more demanding phase cancellation approach can. Real Time Feedback Cancellation™ is a patented feature found on Unitron Hearing's Unison™, Conversa™, and Liason™ products.

DIGITAL COMBINATIONS OF COMPRESSION

Digital hearing aids are, to a large degree, software driven. Because of this fact, digital hearing aids simply combine all sorts of compression types. Always remember those building blocks of compression discussed earlier in Chapter 5; they are fundamental to understanding compression in both analog and digital hearing aids. Readers of Chapter 5 may recall the left-hand graph shown in Figure 7–6; it shows the way compression is often adjusted, and it is the way that many clinicians understand compression. The compression ratios hinge from a kneepoint that is situated to the left, and over a relatively low-input SPL. Higher compression ratios here result in decreased gain.

Readers of Chapter 6, where we discussed multi-channel and programmable hearing aids, will also recall the right-hand graph shown in Figure 7–6. It shows the way compression began to be adjusted with the advent of those high-end two-channel analog hearing aids of the late 80s and 90s. As we have seen, OHC damage, resultant loudness growth requirements, and WDRC really played a big part of hearing aid development 10 years ago. Notice the compression ratios hinge from a kneepoint that is situated to the right, and over a relatively high-input SPL. Here, a higher compression ratio results in *increased* gain.

Digital hearing aids often combine both of these types of kneepoints, so that the input/output graph now has two kneepoints (Figure 7–7). In some digital hearing aids, even more kneepoints can be specified. In Figure 7–7, maximum gain occurs below the left-most kneepoint. Here, the gain is linear. Even greater than linear gain can also occur; this is called "expansion," and it will be covered next in this chapter. WDRC, with its low compression ratio, occurs between the two kneepoints. Above the right-most kneepoint, output-limiting compression occurs with its high compression ratio. The purpose here is to limit the MPO for high input sound levels.

Different Ways of Adjusting Compression

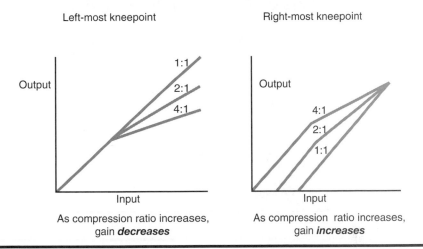

Left-most kneepoint

1:1
2:1
4:1

Output

Input

As compression ratio increases,
gain *decreases*

Right-most kneepoint

Output

4:1
2:1
1:1

Input

As compression ratio increases,
gain *increases*

FIGURE 7–6 The left panel shows compression adjustments in the way that most clinicians conceive of them. When hinging from a left-most kneepoint, linear (1:1) gain implies greatest gain. Increased compression ratios imply progressively less gain. The right panel shows compression as it originally became available with high-end multi-channel analog hearing aids of the mid to late 1990s. This type of compression adjustment was based on the model of normal loudness growth. With compression hinging from the right-most kneepoint, linear gain is actually the least amount of gain offered, while increased compression ratios imply increased gain. The objective here was to approximate normal loudness growth with increased compression ratios. Today's digital hearing aids commonly utilize both of these ways of adjusting compression.

Most manufacturers provide software for the fitting of their high-end hearing aids, including their digital hearing aids. Input/output graphs sometimes comprise a section of the fitting software, and the results of kneepoint and compression ratio adjustments can be seen. On digital hearing aids, two or more kneepoints can often be separately and independently adjusted, which in turn, adjusts the compression ratios.

Raising the left-most kneepoint vertically increases the compression ratio for soft-moderate level input sounds, which increases the gain for these sounds (Figure 7–8). This accomplishes the same thing as increasing the compression ratio as shown in the right panel of Figure 7-6. Moving the left-most TK to the left does nothing to the compression ratio itself, but it does have the effect of increasing the gain for very soft input sound levels. This accomplishes the same thing as moving the TK control, as discussed in Chapter 5.

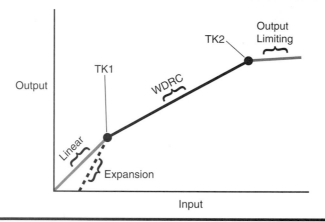

Two Kneepoints, with Linear, WDRC, Output Limiting

FIGURE 7–7 Digital hearing aid fitting software commonly enables clinicians to visualize input/output graphs showing two (or more) kneepoints. Each kneepoint can be adjusted both vertically and horizontally, to best meet the needs of the client. Linear gain takes place below the left-most kneepoint; WDRC occurs between the two kneepoints, while output limiting compression occurs to the right of the right-most kneepoint. In many digital hearing aids, expansion is also offered. Expansion provides greater than linear gain, and it occurs below the left-most kneepoint.

Raising the right-most TK vertically has the effect of decreasing the compression ratio (Figure 7–9). This increases the gain, but only for the more intense sound inputs the MPO of the hearing aid; the most obvious effect is to increase the MPO. Moving the right-most TK to the right, again has no effect on the compression ratio, but it does increase the gain for the most intense input sounds. These two adjustments of the right-most TK (raising it vertically or moving it horizontally) together accomplish the same thing as adjusting the MPO with the output limiting compression control, as discussed earlier in Chapter 5. The digital difference here is that these two adjustments can be done separately, whereas in analog hearing aid circuits, they both happened simultaneously.

Some digital hearing aids utilize multi-kneepoint input/output functions, and their stated purposes proposed by the manufacturers of these hearing aids are quite interesting. Figure 7-10 shows an example of such an input/output function. The literature for Oticon's Syncro™ hearing aid, for example, states the reasoning for their input/output function as follows. Expansion (to be described in the next section), for example, is called "soft squelch," and it appears below the first or left-most kneepoint at around 25 dB SPL. The purpose is to reduce annoying audible internal hearing aid noise that is below the intensity of typical speech. WDRC appears between the 1st and 2nd kneepoints (25 dB to 45 dB SPL), and its

Raise Left TK Vertically...

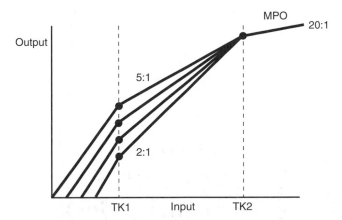

• *Increases compression ration*
• *Increases gain for soft/mid-level inputs*

FIGURE 7–8   The left-most kneepoint can be adjusted vertically and/or horizontally. An increased WDRC ratio results from raising this kneepoint (since the compression here hinges from the right-most kneepoint). This serves to increase the gain for soft- to mid- level input intensity sounds. If the same kneepoint were to be moved horizontally to the left, this would do nothing to the compression ratio itself, but it would have the effect of increasing the gain for very soft input sound levels.

purpose is to increase audibility of soft speech, and also, to hear softer sounds that are a further distance away. The compression ratio is increased between the 2nd and 3rd kneepoints (45 dB and 65 dB SPL), thus providing less gain for these inputs. The stated reason is because listening conditions are supposedly quite good between these levels. From 65 dB to about 80 dB SPL, the gain is again linear! At these levels, speech and noise are commonly mixed together, and people generally prefer increased gain in these situations, so as to hear speech better in these more difficult listening situations. Past 80 dB SPL inputs, the compression ratio is dramatically increased in order to limit the MPO.

The point here is not whether Oticon is right or wrong in its stated objectives; rather, clinicians should be aware that the digital hearing aid manufacturing sector is highly innovative. To increase identification and marketability, twists of all natures and kinds are provided. At times, a feature can be created out of a realization of a flaw in the design! The author recalls one manufacturer noticing a rather rounded looking kneepoint in the input/output graph of one of its older products. When the concept of "curvilinear" compression appeared (in the mid 1990s), this product began to be advertised and promoted as providing curvilinear compression. Whether it did or not was one thing; the point is that the concept of curvilinear compression did not even exist at the time when

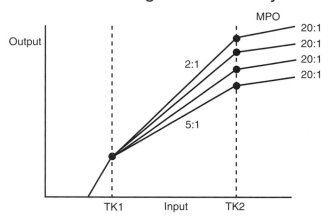

Raise Right TK Vertically...

- •Compression ratio decreases
- •Gain increases for intense input levels

FIGURE 7–9   The right-most kneepoint can also be adjusted vertically and/or horizontally. An increased MPO results from raising this kneepoint (since the compression here hinges from the left-most kneepoint). This serves to increase the gain for mid to intense input intensity sounds. If the same kneepoint were to be moved horizontally to the right, this would again do nothing to the compression ratio itself, but it would have the effect of increasing the gain for intense levels.

the product was created! Sometimes, when one actually finds out what some touted feature in fact does, the name it has been given has very little to do with the function the feature does. Like any good consumer, clinicians should make it their business to become knowledgeable of the products manufacturers provide.

Dynamic Compression Characteristics in Digital Hearing Aids

Digital hearing aids also uniquely implement various types of *dynamic* compression characteristics. As we discussed in Chapter 5, there are many possible variations of attack/release times, fixed or adaptive. In the beginning of the digital era, the Widex Senso™ utilized AVC with its long attack/release times; on the other hand, Oticon's DigiFocus™ utilized syllabic detection, which is the opposite (short attack/release times). Today, most digital hearing aid fitting software tends to offer two types for clinicians to choose from: syllabic compression and average detection. Recall from Chapter 5 that syllabic compression is most successfully used along with low-frequency WDRC or BILL; average detection provides adaptive attack and adaptive release times and has no specified frequency

A Multi-Kneepoint Input/Output Graph

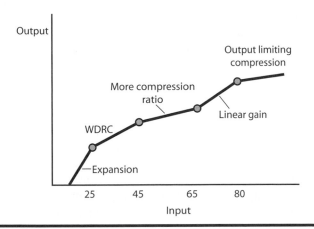

FIGURE 7–10   The software for fitting many digital hearing aids often shows input/output graphs that have more than two kneepoints. Each can be adjusted by the software, or they can be automatically set to a "best-fit" as determined by the fitting software. Below the left-most kneepoint, either linear gain or expansion (commonly called "soft noise squelch") can be selected. Only expansion is shown on this figure. Linear gain, of course, would be a 45° angle.

of usage. Many quick-fit options of digital hearing aids default to the use of syllabic compression for the low-frequency channels and average detection for the high-frequency channels.

As can be seen, many manipulations are possible with digital hearing aids. Clinicians can take comfort from fears of too much freedom; the same fitting software that offers these graphs for adjustment also hides them during "quick fit" options. Furthermore, many manufacturers provide advice, guidance, and fitting solutions on their fitting software.

Adaptive Dynamic Range Optimization (ADRO™)

As we have seen in Chapter 5, and also here in this chapter on digital hearing aids, many facets of compression—kneepoints, ratios, and attack/release times—can be combined together. Add to this, the concept of different compression combinations across different channels in digital hearing aids, and the complexity of compression possibilities balloons even more. In the last few years, a digital alternative to the typical array of compression adjustment parameters has appeared; this method of signal processing is called Adaptive Dynamic Range Optimization (ADRO™). ADRO processing began with usage in cochlear implants and, later on, became a digital algorithm for use in hearing aids (Blamey, Martin, & Fiket, 2004).

With typical compression, the gain is normally adjusted according to fixed rules of input and output, for example, fixed kneepoints, ratios, and selected types of attack/release times. With ADRO, on the other hand, the gain is adjusted very differently (Fortune, 2005). Aided outputs are sampled from the listening environment over several seconds of time, and plotted as a statistical distribution. The statistical distribution of output samples is constantly updated of course, with additional changes that normally occur in the listening environment.

The constantly changing statistical distribution of aided output samples is subjected to two preset, fixed rules or boundaries that apply to the aided outputs; namely, an Audibility criterion of 30% and a Comfort criterion of 90%. The Audibility criterion specifies that up to (and no more than) 30% of all aided outputs can be below some predetermined output level. For any particular client, this predetermined output level should be soft but still audible. The Comfort criterion specifies that at least 90% of all aided outputs must be less than some higher predetermined output level. For the same particular client, this second predetermined output level should be one that is loud, but not uncomfortably loud.

With changes to the listening environment, the statistical distribution of aided output levels will slide to lower or higher intensities, and sometimes then, the rules or criteria will necessarily need to be enforced. If, for example, more than 10% of aided outputs become higher than the Comfort criterion, the gain is automatically reduced until the aided outputs "obey" the rule. If, on the other hand, more than 30% of aided outputs fall below the Audibility criterion, the gain is accordingly increased.

Signal processing with ADRO results in rather slow changes to gain over time; either 3 dB or 6 dB/second, depending on the preferences of the aided listener. As such, ADRO could be said to provide a type of *automatic volume control*, as mentioned earlier in Chapter 5. Here, however, the reader must be cautious not to interpret ADRO simply as compression with slow attack/release times. In his very readable article on ADRO, Fortune (2005) reminds us that typical compression adjusts gain according to its preset kneepoints and ratios, and that it does so *for all changes to input levels*. In contrast, ADRO waits until the output levels fall below the Audibility criterion or exceed the Comfort criterion; only when these "violations" occur, does ADRO call for adjustments to the gain.

The "rub" of ADRO is that it changes gain only when the aided output disobeys the two criteria of Audibility and Comfort. Unlike typical compression, ADRO thus offers a *range* of gain for any one specific input level. Recall that the goal of ADRO is to maintain aided outputs so that they sit between the Audibility and the Comfort criteria. Fortune (2005) offers another description for ADRO; linear gain is given when the aided outputs meet the two criteria, while compression is given when either criteria is violated. Such a default to linear gain offers yet another advantage for clarity of speech cues: Recall in Chapter 5 where we discussed the reasoning that WDRC, which provides greatest gain for soft sounds and less gain for moderately intense sounds, can compromise the differences between the "peaks" and valleys" of the speech waveform

(Kuk, 1999). Since ADRO applies linear gain more often, provided the outputs meet the two criteria, this degradation of the speech waveform becomes less of a threat to important speech cues. The reader is invited to read further on this exciting new digital algorithm for compression.

EXPANSION

Expansion is the opposite of compression. On the basis of everything discussed so far, one might wonder when this would ever be of use. Basically, expansion is a way to reduce internal microphone and amplifier noise that sometimes becomes audible to the listener in quiet, especially those who have good low-frequency hearing. Expansion actually serves to reduce the gain for very soft input sounds (e.g., below 40 dB SPL), and then rapidly increasing the gain as inputs increase, up until the first kneepoint of compression. Expansion was actually offered on an analog circuit produced by Gennum, the DynamEQIII™, but the advent of digital technology precluded its use in hearing aids. Today, most digital hearing aids offer expansion.

Here's how and why it works: Figure 7-11 shows expansion on an input/output graph, as it is superimposed on typical WDRC, offered by some fictitious hearing aid. The vertical output line is extended downward on this figure, further than usual, in order to show where the function of expansion would terminate. Note that the gain for 0 dB SPL input would be nothing, so the output would also be 0 dB SPL. Note also, how the gain dramatically increases, however, as the inputs increase, up until the kneepoint shown here. With *greater* than 1:1 linear gain, expansion thus provides maximum gain at (and only at) the left-most kneepoint seen in most input/output graphs. Hopefully, this left-most, lower kneepoint is set at an input level typical to soft conversational speech, because soft speech is then what gets the greatest amount of gain for the listener. Expansion in digital hearing aids commonly offers expansion ratios of 1:5, 1:75, or 1:2. With a 1:2 compression ratio, for example, for each added decibel of input, there would be two decibels of added output!

As mentioned earlier, expansion is mainly used to reduce the gain for soft, internal microphone and amplifier noise. The left graph of Figure 7-12 shows an input/output graph for a typical WDRC hearing aid. This is essentially the same graph for the same fictitious WDRC hearing aid as that shown on Figure 7-11; however, the vertical output line is no longer extended below the horizontal input line. On the left graph, straight WDRC without the use of expansion would provide 40 dB of linear gain below the knee point. The WDRC here provides a 2:1 compression ratio. Again, the solid line extending downward to the left of the kneepoint shows expansion when used with this WDRC hearing aid. The expansion in this example gives a 1:2 input/output ratio. It is important to note that expansion is always offered only below the left-most kneepoint. Its purpose is to give more than linear gain, but only for very soft inputs.

Here's the rub with expansion; for *really* soft inputs, like 10 dB to 20 dB SPL, there is very little gain. In the example shown in Figure 7-12, there is a dramatic,

Expansion

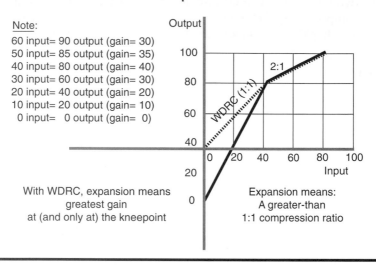

Note:
60 input= 90 output (gain= 30)
50 input= 85 output (gain= 35)
40 input= 80 output (gain= 40)
30 input= 60 output (gain= 30)
20 input= 40 output (gain= 20)
10 input= 20 output (gain= 10)
 0 input= 0 output (gain= 0)

With WDRC, expansion means
greatest gain
at (and only at) the kneepoint

Expansion means:
A greater-than
1:1 compression ratio

FIGURE 7–11 Expansion is the opposite of compression. Unlike WDRC, it provides greater than linear gain for inputs that are below the kneepoint of compression. Note in this example, how the gain increases as the inputs increase from 0 dB SPL to 40 dB SPL; for increasing inputs beyond the kneepoint, the gain once again decreases. When WDRC is used along with expansion, the greatest gain is delivered at (and only at) the left-most kneepoint of compression.

greater-than-linear increase of gain however, as the input intensities increase up to the kneepoint set at 40 dB SPL. Past the kneepoint, the hearing aid goes into compression. The right graph on Figure 7–12 shows the very same hearing aid, but this time the vertical axis shows gain and not output. Note that the WDRC hearing aid in this example is providing a steady amount (40 dB) of gain for all inputs below the kneepoint. When the same hearing aid uses expansion, however, there is less gain for the really soft input sounds of 0 dB to 20 dB SPL. Again, with expansion, the maximum gain is seen *at, and only at*, the kneepoint of compression. The gain increases as input sound levels increase up to the kneepoint, and then as compression kicks in, the gain is once again reduced. WDRC hearing aids that use expansion and have a kneepoint of around 40 dB, provide maximum gain for soft sounds of speech.

People who complain that their WDRC hearing aids make a "hissing" sound in quiet are apt to appreciate the benefits of expansion. These people also most likely have good low-frequency hearing. Recall from Chapter 5 that the focus of WDRC hearing aids is to "lift the floor" of hearing sensitivity, to imitate the OHCs, and to amplify soft sounds by a lot and loud sounds by little or nothing at all. Clinicians can counsel Mrs. McGillicudy that the hearing aid is meant to imitate the OHCs, etc. But if she has good hearing in the low frequencies, she may still say, "I hate my hearing aid in quiet because it makes a hissing sound." This is because WDRC by itself is "trying too hard" to imitate OHCs. In really quiet

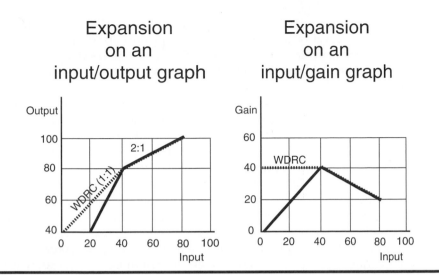

FIGURE 7–12 The left panel shows expansion on an input/output graph. The example here is the same as that shown in Figure 7-10. The gain of the WDRC hearing aid here in this example is 40 dB. WDRC (dotted line) provides linear gain for soft inputs below the kneepoint. Expansion is shown as the solid line below the kneepoint. Note that its function is steeper than the typical 45° angle function of linear gain. The right panel shows the same expansion and WDRC, only this time, they are displayed on an input/gain graph. WDRC provide a constant (linear) amount of gain for all inputs below the kneepoint; once past (to the right of) the kneepoint, the gain drops off due to compression. In comparison, expansion provides increased gain with increased input levels up until the kneepoint. Again, with expansion, the greatest gain is only at the first kneepoint of compression. Hopefully, this maximal gain is provided for soft speech inputs.

surroundings, it will provide maximum gain, and her good low-frequency hearing will pick up unwanted internal microphone and amplifier noise. Expansion thus acts like an internal noise squelch feature. In fact, some of the digital hearing aid literature calls expansion a "soft squelch" feature. It is useful mostly for those who have mild-moderate SNHL, and would otherwise benefit from WDRC.

DIGITAL NOISE REDUCTION (DNR) METHODS

We all (even those with normal hearing) have increased difficulty listening to speech in background noise. As discussed earlier in Chapters 1 and 3, the problem is even worse for those with SNHL. This is why the promise of digital noise reduction (DNR) was looked at with so much hope, when it first came out in digital hearing aids with the Widex Senso™ in 1997. It's not that analog circuitry cannot accomplish DNR; rather, as we have seen earlier, DSP is far more flexible because it is based on numerical manipulations. DSP therefore handles DNR much better. However, the promise of DNR in hearing aids did not necessarily turn out as planned. This is not because present DSP algorithms are so poor;

rather, it is because speech and noise sounds are so inextricably mixed together. The complete removal of background noise from the mixed up speech and noise is easier said than done. The purpose of this section is to explain how DNR works in digital hearing aids. The clinical benefits of DNR will be discussed in Chapter 8.

DNR has been utilized in the military, the telecommunications industry, etc. (Schum, 2003a). Various types will be explained below. With *spectral subtraction*, the spectrum of the speech and the background noise mixed together is measured. The spectrum of the noise itself is estimated *as closely as possible*, and this spectrum of noise is then subtracted from the spectrum of the speech mixed with the noise (Chabries & Bray, 2002; Schum, 2003b). Sometimes, the spectrum of noise is measured during a pause in conversation, and this is subtracted from the speech-plus-noise spectrum (Levitt, 2001). The desired end effect is to remove as much of the noise as possible, without at the same time removing too much of the speech. The main limitation with this approach is the width of the noise spectrum, and how much this width intersects with that of the normal speech spectrum. If the noise spectrum is very narrow, or has several narrow bandwidths, then subtracting this from the total speech and noise spectrum will not remove many of the speech frequencies. As is the case with most annoying or bothersome noise interference, there will more than likely be some intersection between the spectrum of the noise and the spectrum of speech. Of course, there will then be some removal of speech frequencies with spectral subtraction; the point here is to remove as few of the speech frequencies as possible.

Much interfering noise, like that of machinery, or even that of background cafeteria noise has a fairly wide bandwidth. Subtracting this wide bandwidth from the total spectrum of the noise plus the speech of interest will necessarily remove much of the spectrum of the speech of interest.

Phase cancellation is a more advanced approach for DNR (Schum 2003a). In this approach, the *exact waveform* of the interfering noise—not simply its frequency spectrum—must be measured. If this can be done, then the phase of the noise waveform is flipped 180° in phase, so that it can be added and, therefore, cancelled out. This is the type DNR used in high-end noise-reduction headphones. In this case, the speech signal of interest is coming straight from the headphone transducer into the ear canal. The interfering noise, on the other hand, is arriving from the sound field outside of the headphone. Phase cancellation can be readily accomplished with these headphones because nearly the exact waveform of the noise can be captured outside of the headphone, just before it enters the ear. When the phase is digitally reversed so that it is opposite in phase, it can then be added from the headphone to the existing speech and the noise inside the ear canal.

As Schum (2003b) points out, digital hearing aids do not have this luxury, because the sound picked up by the hearing aid microphone already has both the speech and the noise! The noise waveform cannot be separately and accurately measured in this situation. As a result, it cannot be reversed in phase so as to cleanly delete it from the speech and noise waveform.

Other approaches to DNR can also be made. Instead of trying to delete or remove the noise from speech, the speech itself can be enhanced. Some research has tried "*spectral enhancement*," although they did it with analog technology available to them at the time (Stone & Moore, 1992). It did not meet with much success. In this method, a DSP algorithm attempts to recognize spectral speech cues amidst the background noise, and enhance these, so as to improve the recognition of speech in the noise. Peaks in the spectrum of speech largely contain the cues for understanding or recognizing speech. It is well known that a spectrum of speech in background noise shows that the "valleys" between the peaks of speech are filled with noise, thus, making the peaks less prominent against or compared to the valleys. Those with SNHL have an especially difficult time discerning the peaks of speech from the valleys when they are filled with noise and, therefore, are greatly affected by background noise when trying to listen to speech. The idea behind spectral enhancement is to deliberately increase the intensity of the peaks and troughs in the speech-plus-noise spectrum and to, thus, make the speech more easily recognizable.

The trouble with this approach, says Schum (2003b), is that low-frequency, tonal vowel formants are normally more intense than the soft non-tonal noises of high-frequency unvoiced consonants. It is easier for digital algorithms to spectrally enhance the peak-to-valley spectral content of the vowels than for high-frequency unvoiced consonants. Yet it is precisely these high-frequency speech sounds that are commonly the most difficult for those with SNHL to hear!

In their experiment with spectral enhancement, Stone and Moore (1992) used an analog filter bank composed of 16 channels. Various channels among the 16 were used to increase the intensity of the speech peaks, depending on the frequencies present in the speech input sounds. A total of 10 subjects with mild-to-moderate SNHL were tested for their speech reception ability in the presence of continuous background noise. In one experiment, subjects wore their own hearing aids, most of which were linear. The background noise was presented at two different levels (44 dB and 64 dB SPL), and the speech was presented at a level that was 3 dB more intense than these background noise levels. In another experiment, the subjects did not wear their hearing aids; instead, the stimuli were given high-frequency emphasis so as to imitate the function of their own hearing aids. In the second experiment, the subjects adjusted the level of the background noise to match levels they normally found to be comfortable in their everyday lives. Speech intelligibility did not improve for Moore's subjects, but in some cases, it became worse! The second experiment, however, did show that they did have a *subjective* impression that speech stood out better against background noise.

Another attempt at enhancing speech relative to background noise is *speech synthesis* (Schum, 2003b). In this approach, the DSP algorithm again tries to detect speech cues in background noise; this time, however, synthesized speech sounds are *added* to the detected speech sounds in order to enhance their recognition. This may require a collection of previously stored speech sounds that sound like the detected speech cues, and the subsequent addition of these to the detected speech cues.

The synthesized speech method of speech enhancement also comes with its problems. If the background noise is competing speech, this can wreak some havoc with this approach. So also does the required complexity of a digital algorithm that can accurately accomplish this, especially for soft, transient unvoiced speech sounds. Furthermore, Schum (2003b) points out that the resultant speech can sound quite unnatural.

Digital Noise Reduction (DNR) in Digital Hearing Aids

In some digital hearing aids, a form of spectral subtraction has been used as an algorithm for DNR (Bray & Nilsson, 2000). In other digital hearing aids, some speech enhancement has also been utilized as an algorithm. Phase cancellation is actually used in some digital algorithms for feedback reduction and it is also used in directional microphones. We have already briefly looked at feedback reduction in this chapter. More on directional microphones is covered in the next chapter. Let's look more specifically at how DNR and speech enhancement are employed in today's digital hearing aids.

Recall that spectral subtraction is an actual subtraction of the noise spectrum from the noise-plus-speech spectrum. This real subtraction is not done to accomplish DNR in digital hearing aids because far too much speech information would be lost. We cannot forget that those who wear hearing aids have hearing loss and so, a further loss of the redundancy of speech acoustics is definitely not what we want to provide.

In order to accomplish a weaker degree of spectral subtraction, DNR algorithms in digital hearing aids attempt to characterize the acoustic properties of speech versus those of noise. This is done to identify the presence of speech versus noise in each band or channel (group of bands) of the hearing aid. If a band or channel is found to have an undue amount of noise, the gain in that band or channel is reduced, usually by some 5 dB to 20 dB. The technique used to detect whether a channel contains mostly speech or noise inputs is the use of amplitude modulation detection and, to a lesser degree, frequency modulation detection.

We have already noted in Chapter 4 that average, ongoing conversational speech spoken in quiet has a dynamic range (peak-to-peak amplitude) of about 30 dB. So also, speech spoke in quiet has "peak-to-valley" dips or changes in intensity, that are about 15 dB "deep" (Schum, 2003b). These are the amplitude modulations of speech. In addition, these modulations occur at a frequency of about 3 to 10 times per second (3–10 Hz). According to Mueller and Ricketts (2005), syllables are about 75 to 150 milliseconds in length, these together with the pauses in speech result in about 4 to 6 modulations per second. On the other hand, noises typical to our usual listening environments have a lot less fluctuations in intensity over time. These acoustic properties, unique to speech, are what most DNR algorithms seize upon in order to identify speech versus noise in each band or channel of the digital hearing aid.

Another thing to be considered is the shrunken depth of amplitude modulations when speech is embedded in noise. If and when this happens, it

Noise Reduction
Most Digital Hearing Aids Use It...

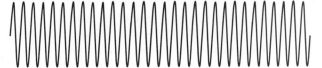

Sounds that don't change in intensity are reduced

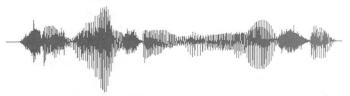

Sounds that don't change in intensity (speech)
are not reduced

FIGURE 7–13   The waveform of a pure tone is shown in the top panel, and the waveform for typical speech is shown in the bottom panel. For both panels, the vertical axis thus represents amplitude, and the horizontal axis represents time. Noise, such as that of a fan or air conditioner, can be construed as fairly steady in intensity over time, much like the pure tone depicted here. Speech, on the other hand, rapidly fluctuates in intensity over time. This difference in amplitude modulation is what DNR algorithms use to determine if the incoming signal input is speech or noise.

becomes more difficult for the DNR algorithm to determine what constitutes speech and what constitutes noise. In any case, some decision rule is adopted for use by the DNR algorithm to determine the ratio of modulation that constitutes speech. In most digital hearing aids, the same gain is applied to a channel regardless if speech alone is present in that channel or if mostly speech and some noise are present (Mueller & Ricketts, 2005). This is done to prevent an excessive loss in audibility. Many digital hearing aids also produce progressively less and less gain in a channel as the sound becomes less and less modulated (more and more steady-state).

DNR algorithms take some time to maximally reduce the gain (by 5 dB to 20 dB) in frequency bands or channels where noise is sensed. According to Mueller and Ricketts (2005), this time can vary anywhere from 2 seconds to 20 seconds, depending on the specific digital hearing aid model and manufacturer. The time it takes to return to original gain again can be quick (5 milliseconds) to a few seconds.

Let's look at typical DNR, as seen in Figure 7-13. Two sounds are shown here; the top sound is steady in intensity over time, while the bottom sound fluctuates much more in intensity over time (time is shown on the horizontal axis, and intensity is shown on the vertical axis). The sinusoid pattern of the top sound is really that typical to a pure tone, which in this case is steady in intensity over time. In a similar way, noise is also assumed by the DNR algorithm to be steady in intensity over time, especially when compared to the fluctuations of speech, shown in the bottom panel. Think of the steady, constant hum of an air conditioner or a fan. One may ask, "What about background *speech* that you don't want to hear? That, too, may be considered as noise." Now is the time to think about the English alliterations "babble" or "hubbub," because these also suggest that the intensity of background speech is relatively steady in intensity over time.

Compare the relatively *steady* intensity of background cocktail party speech (considered as "noise" by the DNR algorithm) to the *fluctuating* intensity of speech spoken by a person right in front. It is not easy for most of us to abstractly think about the acoustics of speech as separate from the meaning of speech, but the acoustics of speech themselves are truly quite unique. As mentioned in Chapter 3, the actual acoustic pops, fizzes, stops, and sputters of speech are difficult to appreciate unless one goes out and listens to a language he/she cannot understand. In that situation, all meaning becomes stripped (dogs and cats must be laughing their heads off at us).

Unlike noise, the intensity of speech is very unevenly distributed. As mentioned already back in Chapter 4, the nonparametric distribution of speech intensity is the reason its *mean* intensity is not situated in the middle of its general 30 dB *range* of intensity. There, we discussed that speech (in contrast to most background noises) has an abnormal statistical distribution of intensity levels. This is why Figures 4–5 and 4–6 do not show the mean of long-term speech intensity to be located right in the very center of the range of speech intensity.

It is precisely this unique fluctuation in input sounds that the digital noise reduction algorithm determines must be speech; if so, the gain is left alone and not reduced. It's the steady-state intensity sounds that the digital noise reduction algorithms are searching for. If such is found in any frequency band or channel, the mission for DNR is to drop the gain in that band or channel by some 5 dB to 20 dB. The actual amount of gain reduction depends on the manufacturer and the choices you have entered on the fitting software.

Come to think of it, however, with a voice kept at a constant intensity, like humming a tone, the DNR algorithm just might consider that to be noise, and reduce the gain accordingly. This is exactly what some digital hearing software has taken into account, when fitting clients who might want a program for listening to music. In this situation, the DNR algorithm is usually shut off. For optimal DNR, in other words, for the very least reduction in speech information, two things would have to be the case: (1) the DNR algorithm would operate in each of many narrow frequency bands in a digital hearing aid, and (2) a very narrow band of noise would enter the microphone of the hearing aid. This optimal situation would result in a 5 dB to 20 dB gain reduction over a very narrow frequency band, or small amount, of speech. As most can appreciate, however, this is most often not the case. Indeed, most noise entering the hearing aid has a fairly broad frequency spectrum. Furthermore, the amplitude and frequency characteristics of background speech hubbub can be fairly close to those of the speech of interest, and this only serves to complicate the task of DNR (Chabries & Bray, 2002).

There is a lot of variation in DNR effectiveness among the various manufacturers of digital hearing aids that use it (Mueller & Ricketts, 2005). Research mentioned by those authors states that there is one DNR algorithm that is better than another at providing unattenuated gain for speech across the whole audiometric frequency range of interest; the same DNR reduces the gain for steady-state noise, albeit by somewhat different amounts across the same frequency range. In comparison, another DNR algorithm provides some low-frequency gain reduction even for speech; the same DNR algorithm provides still more low-frequency gain reduction for noise. Both of these DNR algorithms provide a gain reduction for music that is between those provided for speech and for noise.

An Exception to Typical DNR

The generally accepted conventional wisdom today is that there is no objective benefit for improved speech reception in background noise is. There is, however, a small but notable exception to this general finding, and that is offered in a patented DSP technique called *Personalized Noise Reduction*™, in the digital products manufactured by Sonic Innovations (Bray & Nilsson, 2000). Their DNR is also based on spectral subtraction, but it is uniquely coupled with fast, narrow-band compression. The attack/release times are symmetrical. These are about 35 milliseconds in the low-frequency bands (we will call them channels), down to less than 5 milliseconds in the high-frequency channels. Their Natura™ and Conforma™ digital products each have nine channels. Their newest digital product, the Innova™, has the same DNR system working in 16 channels. The Personalized Noise Reduction™ can be programmed to reduce the gain in channels by a maximum amount of 6, or 12, or 18 dB, depending on the degree of one's hearing loss. The DNR begins 2 seconds after the onset of the noise, and takes 5 seconds to provide maximum gain reduction for any channels where noise is sensed. The SNR is calculated for each channel in real time, and greater DNR is provided for channels where the input SNR is the smallest. When noise is sensed in any channel, a portion of the chosen amount of DNR (6, 12, or 18 dB) will then be applied, depending on the actual SNR found in that channel. So, if a larger DNR (e.g., 18 dB) is chosen, this means the gain with incoming noise will change over a greater intensity range.

After the onset of noise, the DNR takes 2 to 5 seconds to start working; once the DNR is activated, however, the actual gain reduction (that is based on the SNR in each channel) uses the time constants of the fast-acting compression. Again, as the SNR becomes poorer, it is more likely that the gain will be rapidly adjusted between the loud portions of the speech. Due to these relatively fast attack/release times, the DNR does not seem to degrade or otherwise interfere with the rapidly changing acoustic properties of speech.

Speech Enhancement

As mentioned before, digital hearing aids have also utilized algorithms for detecting speech in noise that fall more along the lines of speech enhancement (instead of DNR). These algorithms rely on the identification of acoustic properties (other than modulations) that are unique to speech. One such type of speech enhancement algorithms is called "*comodulation*" (Mueller & Ricketts, 2005) or *synchrony detection*^{TM} (Schum, 2003b). This particular algorithm searches the acoustic environment for the harmonic frequencies of the lowest (fundamental) frequencies of speech (in males about 125 Hz, and in females about 250 Hz). These harmonics of speech are far smaller in amplitude than the fundamental frequencies are. In fact, the dB/octave roll-off for speech leaving the mouth is about -6 dB. If these acoustic properties are found, either in quiet or in and amongst background noise, then more gain with less compression is provided. This added gain is given to both the speech and the background noise. If no such harmonics or speech-like properties are detected, then less gain with more compression is provided. In general, more gain is thus given when speech is present. Schum (2003b) is quick to add that this algorithm is no better at separating noise from speech than typical DNR algorithms, but does tout its virtue in provide more listening comfort in background noise.

Synchrony detection algorithms do their job (provide more gain) when speech is present, while DNR algorithms do theirs (provide less gain) when noise is present. The former speech enhancement algorithm is based on an observation that those wearing hearing aids, who *want* to hear the speech that is spoken in noise, tend to prefer the same or even more gain in noise than they do when listening in quiet. Synchrony Detection^{TM} is used on Oticon's Adapto^{TM} digital hearing aid.

TWO EXAMPLES OF EARLY DIGITAL HEARING AIDS

Now that we have looked at common digital features found in today's digital hearing aids, for historical interest, let's look way back to 1996/1997 to see the salient features of the two earliest digital hearing aids. This way we can see how they each were very different pioneers in the utilization of many of the concepts we have looked at in this chapter and in preceding chapters. The Widex Senso^{TM} was the very first digital hearing aid to hit the market. The author recalls well the scene at the American Academy of Audiology convention in 1997. The biggest advance seen by most clinicians was the presence of digital noise reduction (DNR) in the Senso^{TM}. High hopes were placed for finally addressing the classic "speech-in-noise" problem faced by most people with SNHL.

The Senso^{TM} had three channels with adjustable crossover frequency controls, which adjust the frequency where adjacent channels "meet." These crossover controls enable the channels to be widened or narrowed. The gain can be adjusted separately for each channel, depending on the shape of the hearing loss (where it rises or falls). Each channel had WDRC geared to accomplish normal loudness growth for the listener.

An interesting aspect of the Senso™ was that the threshold kneepoint of compression can be set to as low as 15 dB to 20 dB SPL. In the Senso™, this low kneepoint is associated with a larger-than-usual amount of gain for low-intensity input sounds (expansion!). Widex explained that with analog hearing aids, this low kneepoint could not be utilized because excessive feedback would be generated by the large amount of gain applied to the low-intensity input sounds.

The attack/release times of the Senso™ were long, some several hundreds of milliseconds in length; these relatively long dynamic characteristics are the same as those provided by AVC (see Chapter 5). Long attack/release times were employed by the Senso™, because shorter attack/release times combined with the low kneepoint of compression were not well received by many initial users in their field trials. The dynamic aspects of compression remained relatively slow in a stationary noise environment, but they would speed up if a sudden, intense transient sound occurs (Ludvigsen, 1997).

During the initial fitting of the Senso™, in situ audiometry determined hearing thresholds by emitting complex tones from the hearing aid while it is in the ear of the listener. These are used to determine targets for gain. Widex explained that the advantage of this method is that the results include the effects of the ear mold or the shell of the hearing aid in situ (in place) in the ear.

The Senso™ used the first DNR in hearing aids, based on spectral subtraction. Widex explained it as an ongoing statistical method separately in each of its three channels, whereby every few seconds, the speech and background noise are sampled. The properties of single-talker speech versus background speech babble would be found to be statistically different in their intensity fluctuations over time, and this difference could then be used to determine in which frequency band most background noise is present. The assumption is also made that in loud listening situations, speech is also spoken louder (Ludvigsen, 1997). When a channel sensed that background noise is present, the gain for both the speech and the noise was reduced in that channel. Because speech in noise is normally spoken at a more intense level, the speech would still be audible even though the gain for both the speech and the noise had been reduced. This is good, historically interesting stuff to look back upon. Perhaps the reason the product was called the Senso™ was because it was always sensing if the input was speech or noise.

Oticon's DigiFocus™ came out immediately on the heels of the Senso™. It had seven frequency bands. Unlike those of the Widex Senso™, the crossover frequencies of the DigiFocus™ could not be adjusted; that is, bands adjacent to each other could not be widened or narrowed. Despite being fixed in place, the seven bands each represented a relatively narrow range of frequencies, which permitted a high degree of fitting flexibility for people with difficult-to-fit hearing loss configurations. The DigiFocus™ was the first to divide the seven bands into low- and high-frequency ranges (a low-frequency channel composed of three low-frequency bands and a high-frequency channel composed of four high-frequency bands).

Central to the Oticon DigiFocus™ philosophy was the concept of "Adaptive Speech Alignment," which was *not* a type of DNR. The goal of this stated feature was to provide aided speech that would be as intelligible as possible. The focus was, instead, on accurate and specific frequency shaping with the seven bands, reducing the upwards spread of masking, and providing very different attack/release times for the low-frequency and high-frequency channels.

The low-frequency channel provided BILL, along with the fast attack/release times of syllabic compression. The syllabic compression, along with BILL, was designed to reduce the upward spread of masking of the more intense, low-frequency vowels, which can obliterate softer high-frequency consonantal speech. The high-frequency channel provided output limiting compression, along with slower acting attack/release times (what Oticon called "adaptive gain"). Consistent with output limiting (described in Chapter 5), the gain for the high-frequency channel was essentially linear, with a high kneepoint and high compression ratio, so as to limit the output from exceeding the listener's loudness discomfort levels. The attack times for the high-frequency channel were about 20 ms, with release times that vary from about 230 ms to 320 ms. A hoped-for result was a more uniform aided intensity for all speech sounds for the listener, making the softer consonantal sounds of speech more audible without simultaneously making the normally louder vowel portions of speech too loud. Recall our discussion of BILL in Chapter 5 and its conceptual purpose, namely, to reduce the upwards spread of masking. Most background noise is relatively low in frequency. Furthermore, the vowel sounds of speech are more intense and lower in frequency than the unvoiced consonants. Consider the background noise and vowels of speech as the bull and the unvoiced consonants as delicate pieces of china. The whole purpose of BILL, along with syllabic compression, is to "control the bull in the china shop." The DigiFocus™ was an initial digital implementation of this concept.

The purpose of this brief look back at these two pioneering digital hearing aids was to highlight just how very different philosophies of the day were incorporated into digital form. Over the passage of time, neither one of these has been proven to be correct or better than the other. Consider, for example, the fact that Widex addressed audibility and speech reception with WDRC and DNR while Oticon addressed the same with a very different approach—BILL with syllabic detection. Consider also the AVC (long attack/release times) of the Senso™ versus the opposite—syllabic compression (short attack/release times) of the DigiFocus™. Each was put forth as the best possible option by Widex and Oticon. No one went to jail on account of either one; the jury was (and still is) largely out on this one. Today, some 10 years later, many manufacturers still include various elements from both of these attack/release time strategies on their fitting software.

DIGITAL HEARING AIDS: STATE OF THE ART AND THE FUTURE

One thing that is evident about the various available digital products is that the manufacturers are highly secretive about the specific methods they use. This is understandable, considering the highly competitive nature of the digital hearing aid market. To release details of an actual proprietary DSP circuit core to the general arena of hearing aid manufacturing would be giving away what probably took a lot of time and money to develop. Each manufacturer has developed their own type of circuit that also contains very specific algorithms. Unlike typical analog hearing aids, which are built from parts that are often available to any manufacturer, digital hearing aids are very proprietary in their composition. As mentioned earlier, only the microphone and receivers in digital hearing aids can be similar to those of analog hearing aids. The actual DSP circuit core is quite unique to any one specific digital hearing aid, although manufacturers have been known to sell these to other manufacturers. This happened more when digital hearing aids first appeared than it does now, because some manufacturers did not have their own digital research and development off the ground, but still wanted to "enter the game."

On the receiving end, some clinicians have been frustrated over the complexity of the fitting software when fitting digital hearing aids. As stated elsewhere before in this book, the products are, in some ways, like closed boxes: The manufacturer may know what is going on inside the hearing aid, and clinicians is left to trust that the fitting will be satisfactory for clients. Complexity in fitting software has replaced elegant simplicity. Clinicians' eyes glaze over; no wonder that most of them take this easy route!

In the author's opinion, a return to simplicity in software would be a truly welcome thing. Far too many clinicians take the quick fit option and abandon probe tube microphone (real-ear) measures to verify that the predicted gain or output from the software is indeed taking place with the hearing aid situated in the client's ear. Without real ear verification, we stand in danger of forgetting *how to fit* hearing aids.

In digital fitting software over the past several years, it has been interesting to note the departure from a required knowledge of compression types and other technological features on the part of the clinician, and the trend towards addressing psycho-social issues of the client. Minor software adjustments to compression (and other) settings for most digital products today depend on specific answers to specific psycho-social situations and other various listening conditions. The complexity of some digital hearing aid products, when coupled with this client-based focus, can produce software adjustment queries that lean towards the extreme in specificity. To highlight this point at conference presentations, the author has given this tongue-in-cheek example: "Do you have trouble hearing the preacher every second Sunday, when sitting at a $45°$ angle to the right, in the third pew from the front?"

There is yet another patch of thorns in today's digital hearing aids: Many terms relating specifically to individual digital products are not readily understandable, because they are used nowhere else in the industry. Furthermore, the different manufacturers often give similar features different names! This is very confusing to clinicians, because they simply want to understand the *concepts* behind the features. An early example that comes to mind is "Adaptive Speech Alignment," coined by Oticon, and described earlier with regard to their first digital product—the DigiFocus™. Ostensibly, one would never know that this basically referred to the use of BILL along with syllabic detection. A much more recent example of this is the "channel-free" Symbio by Bernafon; it has been notoriously difficult for hearing health care professionals to digest the distinction between "channel-free" and "single channel." As discussed earlier, that term, has been a "bone to be chewed" by clinicians for a couple of years by now. The good thing here though, is that in getting answers, we are forced to educate ourselves further.

As was mentioned at the outset of this chapter, *clinicians must take the time to listen to the specific digital hearing aids they tend to recommend the most.* It is one thing to be persuaded about the remarkable advances touted on glossy marketing brochures; it is quite another to have that "wow!" effect when listening to a hearing aid. The importance of this cannot be overstated. I recall distinctly meeting a student of mine with a flat, moderately-severe SNHL, who had just acquired a new pair of high-end digital BTEs. Just for fun, I put an old pair of analog output limiting compression BTEs on the student's earmolds, manually set the trimmers at mid positions, and asked the student how those sounded. The student's answer was actually quite humorous: "Wow, where did you get these digital hearing aids? They sound so clean!" In today's complex digital offerings, I sometimes take refuge in Occam's Razor (often attributed to the medieval philosopher, William of Ockham), which posits that, "The simplest explanation is the best one."

Aside from this rather cynical look at the present state of affairs, the bottom line is that clients are, indeed, often highly satisfied with their digital hearing aids, noting that they are an improvement from their old analog hearing aids. In the long run, digital advances we have mentioned generally go a long way to provide increased comfort and audibility for the end user. Digital hearing aids can also provide a notoriously *clean sound* to the end user, without the internal amplifier noise commonly associated with some analog circuitry. It's not that we have everything solved here; there is always room for improvement. Audibility has largely been addressed with compression utilized in yesterday's programmable, multi-channel hearing aids, and in today's digital hearing aids. These developments have allowed us to make advances toward our second endeavor; namely, speech-in-noise problem faced by those with SNHL. For these clients, we must increase the signal-to-noise ratio (SNR). In the next chapter, we will look at two specific ways of dealing with this.

SUMMARY

- Analog hearing aids transduce sound into electricity (by way of the microphone), amplify the electrical current, and then transduce this back into sound (by way of the receiver). For the most part, the microphone and receiver portions of digital hearing aids are still analog. Digital hearing aids differ from their analog counterparts in that they have an A/D converter, a central DSP core, and a D/A converter. Digital hearing aids, thus, transduce sound into electricity, electricity into digits, digits back into electricity, and finally, electricity into sound.

- Open versus closed digital platforms were discussed. Open platforms allow a great amount of flexibility, but a disadvantage is required high-power consumption. Today's digital hearing aids are essentially closed platform; the hardware includes what is necessary to provide benefit to the end user.

- Six features typical to digital hearing aids are: in situ testing, the possibility of including many more than two frequency bands or channels, automatic feedback reduction, combinations of compression types, expansion, and DNR.

- In situ testing enables the testing of audiometric thresholds, and subsequent fitting according to various fitting methods, all while the hearing aid is situated in the client's ear. This overcomes the necessity for transforms from 2 cc coupler data, dB SPL to dB HL, etc.

- Digital hearing aids today commonly have many frequency bands; low-end digital products commonly have fewer bands while high-end products will have more. Channels were defined as combinations of frequency bands that share common digital algorithms.

- Automatic feedback reduction digitally reduces high-frequency peaks in the output frequency response while the hearing aid is being worn. This feature reduces the need for the physical presence of filters, which can easily become clogged up with wax.

- Combinations of compression types discussed in Chapter 5 are commonly found in today's digital hearing aids. For example, linear gain is often provided for soft inputs, WDRC for medium-intensity inputs, and output limiting for high-intensity inputs. It is also fairly common to see input and output compression combined, where input compression will be provided for soft to medium intensity inputs, while output compression is provided for more intense inputs.

- Expansion is the opposite of compression and is provided for very soft inputs below the left-most (lowest) kneepoint. Greatest gain is thereby provided at (and only at) the first kneepoint of compression, which represents the input levels of soft speech. Expansion serves to reduce the gain for extremely soft inputs, thereby reducing audibility of internal microphone and amplifier noise. It is often included in medium-power digital hearing aids for mild-to-moderate SNHL, where linear gain and WDRC are utilized.

- DNR comes in several forms. The most common type samples incoming sounds and determines whether these stay steady in intensity over time or fluctuate rapidly in intensity over time. Steady-state intensity is determined to be noise; the gain in any channel where noise is sensed is reduced by some 5 dB to 20 dB. Another type of DNR discussed was that of speech enhancement, which determines whether the incoming sounds have acoustic properties similar to speech. If harmonics similar to those found in speech are detected, the input is determined to be speech; the gain in any channel where speech is sensed is thus increased and the compression is reduced. Neither of these methods works "better" than the other; they are simply different approaches.

- Two older, first-generation digital products were reviewed, for the purpose of seeing how they each incorporated the features previously discussed. These first two digital hearing aids to appear were the Senso™ from Widex and DigiFocus™ from Oticon.

- Hearing aid manufacturers are intensely competitive. Different names are often given to similar digital features. Their fitting software for digital products has become increasingly complex. Psycho-social situations and other various listening conditions are examined, and the answers to these queries largely determine the settings for the digital products. This approach tends to cut clinicians off from their understanding of the "hows" and "whys" behind the adjustments, and reinforces the impression that the 1990s were indeed the "golden" age of compression.

REVIEW QUESTIONS

1. "Sampling rate" refers to:
   a. the assignment of numbers to digital samples of sound.
   b. how often the digital circuit samples an analog signal.
   c. the ability of a digital circuit to accurately represent sound intensity.
   d. none of the above

2. In digital hearing aids, the term "channel" refers to:
   a. groups of frequency bands that share a digital algorithm.
   b. the basic elemental frequency bandwidths that can be individually adjusted.
   c. steep dB/octave roll-offs found at the sides of the frequency bands.
   d. all of the above

3. Feedback is caused by excessive:
   a. low-frequency peaks in the gain frequency response.
   b. high-frequency peaks in the gain frequency response.
   c. high-frequency peaks in the output frequency response.
   d. low-frequency peaks in the output frequency response.

4. If compression ratios hinge from a left-most kneepoint, higher compression ratios result in:
   a. increased gain.
   b. decreased gain.
   c. no change in gain.
   d. none of the above

5. For many digital hearing aids, the input/output graphs show linear gain and/or expansion:
   a. below (to the left of) the left-most kneepoint.
   b. above (to the right of) the left-most kneepoint.
   c. at the part of the input/output function where WDRC is displayed.
   d. above (to the right of) the right-most kneepoint.

6. On these same input/output graphs, output limiting compression is shown:
   a. below (to the left of) the left-most kneepoint.
   b. above (to the right of) the left-most kneepoint.
   c. at the part of the input/output function where WDRC is displayed.
   d. above (to the right of) the right-most kneepoint.

7. On these same input/output graphs, expansion is shown:
   a. below (to the left of) the left-most kneepoint.
   b. above (to the right of) the left-most kneepoint.
   c. at the part of the input/output function where WDRC is displayed.
   d. above (to the right of) the right-most kneepoint.

8. Expansion typically will have a compression ratio closest to:
   a. 1:1.   c. 1:2.
   b. 2:1.   d. 10:1.

9. DNR assumes that:
   a. noise fluctuates rapidly in intensity over time.
   b. speech is relatively stable in intensity over time.
   c. speech is relatively more intense than background noise.
   d. none of the above

10. DNR algorithms tend to reduce gain in any channel where noise is sensed by some:
    a. 40 dB to 50 dB.   c. 20 dB to 30 dB.
    b. 30 dB to 40 dB.   d. 5 dB to 20 dB.

RECOMMENDED READINGS

Henrickson, L., (2004). *Processing delay in digital hearing aids: Perception and measurement.* Presentation at the American Academy of Audiology, Salt Lake City.

Mueller H, & Ricketts, T. (2005). Digital noise reduction: Much ado about something? *The Hearing Journal, 58*(1), 10-17.

REFERENCES

Auriemo, J., Nielson, K., & Kuk, F. (2003). Using DSP to screen hearing aid component defects. *The Hearing Review, 10*(2): 40-43.

Blamey, P., Martin, L., & Fiket, H. (2004). A digital processing strategy to optimize hearing aids outputs directly. *Journal of The American Academy of Audiology, 15*(10): 716-728.

Bray, V., & Nilsson, M. (2000). Objective test results support benefits of a DSP noise reduction system. *The Hearing Review, 7*(11): 60-65.

Chabries, D., & Bray, V. (2002). Use of DSP techniques to enhance performance of hearing aids in noise. In G. M. Davies (Ed), *Noise reduction in speech applications* (chapter 16). Boca Raton: CRC Press.

Edmonds, J., Staab, W. J., Preves, D., & Yanz, J. (1998). "Open" digital hearing aids: A reality today. *The Hearing Journal, 50*(10): 54-60.

Fortune, T. (2005). What the heck is bionic with ADRO? *The Hearing Review, 12*(7): 30-36.

Hayes, D. (2003). Real-time cancellation system offers advantages for controlling feedback. *The Hearing Journal, 56*(4): 41-46.

Henrickson, L. (2004). *Processing delay in digital hearing aids: Perception and measurement.* Presentation (IC 105) given at the American Academy of Audiology, Salt Lake City.

Kuk, F.K. (1998). Open or closed? Let's weigh the evidence. *The Hearing Journal, 50*(10): 54-60.

Kuk, F. (1999). Hearing aid design considerations for optimally fitting the youngest patients. *The Hearing Journal, 52*(4): 48-55.

Levitt, H. (2001). Noise reduction in hearing aids: A review. *Journal of Rehabilitation Research and Development, 38*(1): 111-121.

Ludvigsen, C. (1997, March). Basic rationale of a DSP hearing instrument. *The Hearing Review, 4*(3): 58-70.

Ludvigsen, C., & Topholm, J. (1997). Fitting a wide range compression hearing instrument using real-ear threshold data: A new strategy. *Hearing Review Supplement* (High Performance Hearing Solutions, Vol. II), 37-39.

Mueller, G., and Ricketts, T. (2005). Digital noise reduction: Much ado about nothing? *The Hearing Journal, 58*(1): 10-17.

Pavlovic, C., Bisgaard, N., & Melanson, J. (1998). The next step: "Open" digital hearing aids. *The Hearing Journal, 50*(5): 65-66.

Schum, D. J. (1998). Open digital platforms: Opportunities and responsibilities. *The Hearing Journal, 51*(1): 44-46.

Schum, D. (2003). Noise reduction via signal processing: (1) Strategies used in other industries. *The Hearing Journal, 56*(5): 27-32.

Schum, D. (2003). Noise reduction in hearing aids: (2) 41.Goals and Strategies. *The hearing Journal, 56*(6): 32-41

Stone, M., & Moore, B. (1992). Spectral enhancements for people with sensorineural hearing impairments: Effects on speech intelligibility and quality. *Journal of Rehabilitation Research and Development. 29*(2): 39-56.

8

Clinical Benefits of Directional Microphones versus Digital Noise Reduction

INTRODUCTION

Cochlear hair cell pathology that causes SNHL necessitates two things: increased audibility and increased signal-to-noise ratio (SNR). We briefly addressed these two objectives earlier, in Chapter 3. It is now time to look at this issue again more closely. As we have discussed in Chapters 1 and 3, outer hair cell damage reduces audibility of sounds below conversational speech because it reduces the amplitude of the traveling wave. The same hair cell damage also reduces the sharpening of the traveling wave, that is, our ability to separate frequencies that are close together. In real-life situations, this implies a greater difficulty separating speech from background noise. Our most self-conscious, speech-focused hearing aid fitting methods and the latest, greatest programmable, multi-channel hearing aids with the most advanced types of compression only address audibility. As can be seen in Figure 8–1, hearing aids that only increase audibility, take a soft messy message . . . and turn it into a louder messy message.

Increasing audibility with hearing aids is thus only a partial solution for those with SNHL. The duty here is only half done. We must also increase the signal-to-noise ratio, or SNR. In this way, those with damaged hair cells can more easily separate speech from background noise. Clinicians have long tried to focus on improving the client's experiences when listening to speech in background noise. Today, two ways to address our clients' classic difficulty of listening to speech in the presence of background noise are directional microphones and digital noise reduction (DNR).

The purpose of this final chapter is twofold. First, we will take a close look at directional microphones, and how they can *objectively* improve the SNR, and thus provide the benefit of improved speech reception in background noise. Second, we will take a close look at the clinical benefits of DNR; with few exceptions, it has been shown to *subjectively* enhance listening comfort for the client in background noise. It must be said at the outset of this chapter that directional

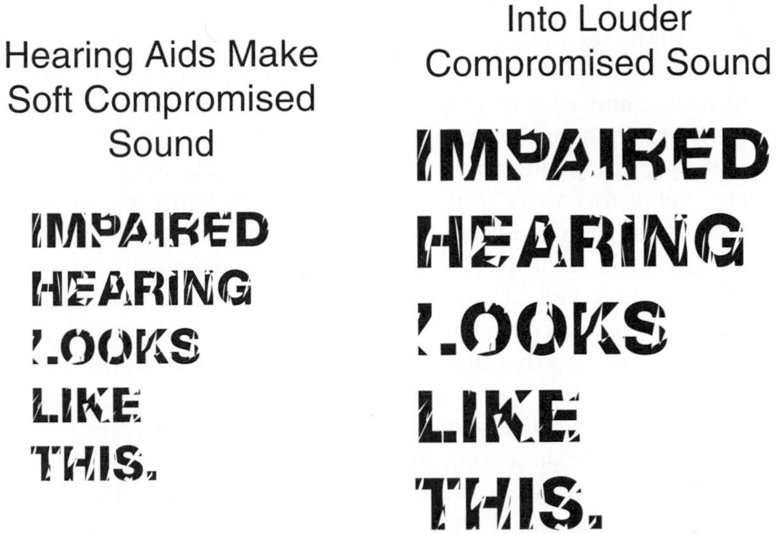

Hearing Aids Make
Soft Compromised
Sound

Into Louder
Compromised Sound

IMPAIRED
HEARING
LOOKS
LIKE
THIS.

IMPAIRED
HEARING
LOOKS
LIKE
THIS.

FIGURE 8–1 For those with SNHL, increasing audibility alone helps the listener hear softer sounds, but this overcomes only part of the problem. Damaged hair cells also result in poorer frequency resolution; namely, a diminished ability to distinguish among frequencies that are close together. This is a big part of the reason that those with SNHL generally have difficulty understanding speech in background noise, even when aided with the best compression available. Aside from increasing audibility, hearing aids should also address this speech-in-noise problem.

microphones improve speech recognition in noise far better than DNR or, for that matter, any other speech enhancement techniques do (Levitt, 2001). Still, both directional microphones and DNR work towards improving listening experiences in background noise. They each simply lend a very different kind of contribution.

DIRECTIONAL MICROPHONES

Like the properties of multi-channel and programmability, directional microphones can be found on both analog and digital hearing aids. In today's digital hearing aids, the microphone(s) and receiver (speaker) are normally analog in form and in function. The truly digital portion in digital hearing aids lies within the digital signal processor (DSP) inside the hearing aid, and this is where the DNR algorithms reside. More will of course be covered on this topic later on. Right now, suffice to say, directional microphones are generally analog. As such, these analog components have been used on yesterday's analog hearing aids as well as on today's digital hearing aids.

Directional microphones have been around for some time; they were invented for use by the military, some 50 years ago! Having been in existence for some 50 years, they have been used in BTEs and on ITEs with sufficient faceplate "real estate" to accommodate them, for about 20 years (Preves, 1997).

The author recalls doing client fittings with analog BTEs that had these earlier directional microphones, during the mid to late 1980s. Usually, the hearing aid had to be ordered as a "directional" model. In a few exceptions, the directionality could be turned on and off with a switch.

Directional microphones in hearing aids were always intended to enhance the SNR by picking up a greater amount of sound from the front of the listener, as compared to sounds that arrive from other angles. Directional microphones do *not* help one tell the direction of sounds, nor do they increase the intensity of sounds coming from the front. Keep in mind that what they actually do is decrease the intensity of sounds coming from the rear, *relative* to sounds coming from the front. In this way, directional microphones can increase the SNR for speech.

Of course, it is assumed that sounds coming from in *front* of the listener are the speech sounds that one *wants* to hear. This may not always be the case, because sometimes the signal (speech) and the noise may both come from the front. In that situation, the directional microphone would do no real good (Bray & Nilsson, 2000). Put it this way, if the speech and the competing noise both come from the same direction, then the directional microphone will have little effect on increasing the SNR. Basically, however, the hoped-for situation is that the speech of interest originates from in front of the listener, while the background noise comes from other directions.

The first generation of directional microphones used in hearing aids did not enjoy much acceptance, mainly because they did not provide for clients the hoped-for benefits. A notable exception to these problems was the Audiozoom™ by Phonak (Kuk, 1996). This was an analog hearing aid model with the best directional microphone of its time. It heralded the comeback of the directional microphone that would take place in a few years (the year after the first digital hearing aids in 1997). In 1992, Everett Koop, the U.S. Surgeon General of the Food and Drug Administration (FDA) put a ban on hearing aid advertisements claiming improved listening in background noise, unless clinical trials could back up this claim. The statistically proven results with Audiozoom™ system won for Phonak, the singular right to advertise that their product truly did improve speech-in-noise performance. Later on, in 1997, the FDA Modernization Act put hearing aids into a different classification; this eliminated the more strict clearance that was previously required for any claims about aided speech in noise (Mueller & Ricketts, 2005).

Killion, M. C., Schulein, R., Christensen, L., Fabry, D., Revit, L., Niquette, P., & Chung, K (1998) addressed the state of directional microphones in general, and took an additional kick at the can; they mention that the "low-tech" solution of cupping one's hand behind the ear to hear better in difficult listening situations provided more benefit than those older directional microphones. Furthermore, a serious oversight on the part of manufacturers at that time was the fact that most of those early directional microphones could not normally be switched off and on at will (Preves, 1997).

Note the years that Preves (1997) and Killion et al. (1998) published their observations; this was just past the time when the first digital hearing aids were appearing in 1997! The DNR on these digital hearing aids did not deliver the hoped-for objective improvement in speech intelligibility. Now was to be the time when directional microphones would enjoy a renaissance, or rebirth. It was almost humorous to watch the manufacturers hurriedly adding directional microphones to their initial digital models. The year 1998 was the year of the second advent of the directional microphone. A notable pioneering push for directionality in the digital age was the D-MIC™ for the ITE, by Etymotic Research (Killion, et al., 1998).

The recent resurgence in directional microphone popularity in the late 1990s was due to a few things: They could be turned on and off by the user, and they became routinely available in full concha ITEs. Furthermore, measurements of improved speech performance in background with directional microphones began to permeate the literature (Killion, 1997a, 1997b; Killion, et al., 1998; Preves, 1998; Roberts & Schulein, 1997). The twofold needs of clients with SNHL, for (1) increased audibility and also (2) increased SNR, were delineated and laid out. Furthermore, directional microphones were now being produced, which "fit the bill," because they were being shown to truly increase the SNR.

Some of the low-cost "second-generation" directional microphones of the late 1990s did have their own problems; they could be quite large. It was a challenge to put them into smaller ITCs because one requirement was that, for greatest effectiveness, the two ports or entries of the directional microphone system had to be at least 10 mm apart. This size requirement collided with the cosmetic urge to keep hearing aids small in size. Furthermore, in comparison to regular, omni-directional microphones, these low-end directional microphones sometimes had a relatively high amount of internal noise. In noisy listening situations, when directionality is most beneficial, it was argued that the internal microphone noise was drowned out (Killion, et al., 1998), but in quiet, the noise was sometimes quite audible to the listener.

How Directional Microphones Work

Microphones are transducers; that is, they change energy from one form into another. In this case, they change sound into electricity. By the way, a receiver is a backwards microphone that changes electricity back into sound again. In the real world (outside of our hearing aids world), this kind of device is usually called a "loudspeaker." Anyway, in a typical hearing aid microphone, sound hits a diaphragm, which causes sound to be changed into electricity (Figure 8–2). If, however, sound were to hit the diaphragm simultaneously from opposite directions, then there would be cancellation. The diaphragm would not be able to vibrate, and the microphone would not be able to do its job.

Omni-directional microphones typically have one door or port for input sounds to enter the microphone. The key thing to note about a *directional* microphone is that they normally have *two* openings or ports for sound to enter (Figures 8–3, 8–4). Note also that the "back" door has a small filter in it. The filter causes incoming sound to be slowed down, because it offers resistance to the passage of sound. First, see what happens when sound comes from the front of the listener (Figure 8–3).

In a Microphone Sound Must Move a Diaphragm

If Sounds Simultaneously Hit Both Sides, The Diaphragm Cannot Move

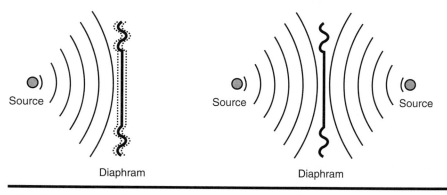

Source   Source   Source

Diaphram   Diaphram

FIGURE 8–2   Microphones are transducers; they change energy from one form into another form. In this case, they change sound into electricity. Incoming sound must be able to vibrate the diaphragm inside the microphone. If sounds simultaneously hit the diaphragm from opposite sides, there is cancellation, and the diaphragm cannot move. This is the basic principle behind directional microphones.

Directional Microphone Function
When Sounds Come From *Front.....*

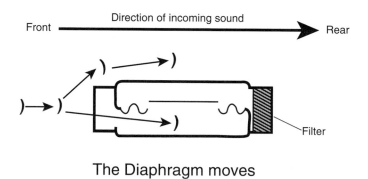

Front   ———— Direction of incoming sound ————▶ Rear

Filter

The Diaphragm moves

FIGURE 8–3   A directional microphone has a delay system in one of its ports. This delay system can be the physical presence of a filter or else it can be electronic. In this figure, the delay is caused by a filter. Sounds coming from the front enter through the front port of the directional microphone, and are able to move the diaphragm.

Directional Microphone Function
When Sounds Come From *Rear.....*

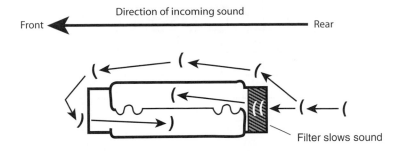

The Diaphragm *cannot* move

FIGURE 8–4   Sounds coming from the rear arrive at the rear port of the directional microphone first. They are delayed (slowed down) by the presence of the filter. The rest of the sound arrives at the front door of the microphone. The delayed incoming sound passing through the rear port filter, and the incoming sound coming through the front port arrive at opposite sides of the diaphragm at the same time. When this happens, there is cancellation, and the diaphragm cannot move.

Figure 8-3 shows sound coming from the front of the listener who is wearing the hearing aid with the directional microphone. Incoming sound enters into the front port of the directional microphone; it vibrates the diaphragm, and the rest of the sound moves on. . . . Now consider an example where sound enters the directional microphone from behind the listener (Figure 8-4). Notice again, that the rear port or doorway has a filter in it. Sound coming from the rear enters into the rear port first, but is slowed down by the filter. The rest of the sound carries on past the rear door, and enters the front door of the directional microphone. Due to the filter in the rear door, which slows the passage of those sounds down, sounds from both the rear and the front hit the diaphragm at the same time, and there is cancellation. This is the basic idea behind directional microphones and shows how they tend to be less sensitive to sounds originating from directions other than the front.

The older, cheaper versions of directional microphones were simple structures with one diaphragm and two ports, as shown in Figures 8-3 and 8-4. In addition, they required almost 10 mm distance between the two ports, which routinely precluded their use in smaller ITE hearing aids. Newer (and more expensive) directional microphones consist of two separate omni-directional microphones situated side by side. These twin omni-directional microphones are often found in higher-end hearing aids. They are sometimes referred to as "dual-microphone processing" (Thompson, 2003). Also, instead of relying on spatial time delays between the sounds arriving at each of the two ports,

Directional Microphones & Hz Response

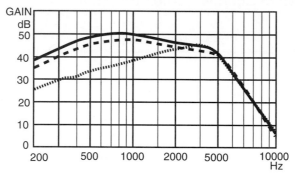

Many directional mics have several positions

Solid Line   • omni-directional
Dashed Line • directional equalized to omni-directional response
Dotted Line • directional with low-cut response

FIGURE 8–5   Directional microphones tend to have a slight drop in the low frequencies in their frequency response. This causes a drop in the overall output frequency response of the hearing aid too. In older, cheaper directional microphones, attempts were made to equalize the directional frequency response so that it was similar to the omni-directional frequency response. This required an increase in entire frequency response of the microphone, along with some filtering of the high frequencies, to best match the omni-directional microphone frequency response. This also, however, tended to increase the noise floor of the equalized directional microphone.

the dual-microphone directional system uses electronic time delays (Mueller & Ricketts, 2000). As a result, the physical spatial distance is less of a factor in determining their effectiveness. They are also known to have a more quiet noise floor than the cheaper, single microphone with two ports. Furthermore, dual-microphone processing enables the directional sensitivity (as seen on "polar plots") to be readily adjusted. This can be achieved with either analog or digital signal processing (Thomson, 2003). On digital hearing aids, even more advanced dual directional microphones have the capacity to change the shape of their polar plots at will. "Adaptive directional" systems on these high-end digital hearing aids offer the additional property of automatically changing polar plot shape, depending on the particular listening environment! More will be discussed on polar plots and adaptive directionality later on.

It should also be recognized that, due to their design, directional microphones tend to cut out low frequencies (Figure 8–5). Low frequencies have longer wavelengths, which bend around objects more than the shorter wavelengths of high frequencies do. As a result, for any particular model of hearing aid, the frequency response of the directional version will show a cut in low frequencies, as compared to the omni-directional version. In fact, this low cut in the microphone's frequency response tends to increase as the two ports of a directional microphone are separated by a distance of less than 10 mm (Thompson, 2003).

Directional microphone systems can be classified according to their complexity (Dittberner, 2003). Both the simpler directional microphone (with one diaphragm and two ports) and the more expensive, quieter directional microphone (consisting of two separate omni-directional microphones placed side by side) are *first-order* directional microphones, because they each have two ports. As such, they are single directional microphones. *Second- and third-order* directional microphone systems consist of two or more directional microphones; these offer even more directionality than first-order directional microphones do. More will be discussed on these later in this chapter.

Directional Microphones: How They are Measured

The benefit of directional microphone for speech intelligibility can be quite easily demonstrated in laboratory test conditions. Figure 8–6 shows four polar plots, which illustrate the sensitivity of a stationary microphone to sounds coming from all different directions. In general, polar plots show patterns of directional sensitivity. The polar plots in Figure 8–6 are idealized; that is, they do not include the real effects of head shadow, sound diffraction, etc. If these factors were included, the resultant polar plots would be more ragged and bumpy in shape (this always does occur for a directional microphone on a hearing aid worn on an ear on the side of one's head).

The omni-directional microphone polar plot is round, showing that it is equally sensitive to sounds coming from all directions. In other words, the omni-directional microphone is no more sensitive to sounds originating from the front than it is to sounds coming from any other directions. Three different types of directional patterns are illustrated by the other three polar plots in Figure 8–6. All of these are equally sensitive to sounds originating from in front of the listener, but they have unequal sensitivity to sounds coming from the other directions.

A numerical quantification can be calculated for any polar plot. This is known as the directional index (DI). The DI for any particular microphone is the ratio of that microphone's sensitivity to frontal sounds than to sounds from all other directions. The frontal sounds are at 0°. The relative sensitivity of that same microphone is then calculated for every other degree of direction. If the microphone is omni-directional, it will have a DI of 0, because it will be no less sensitive to sounds from all other directions. A truly directional microphone, however, should be less sensitive to sounds from other directions.

Take a look at the "cardioid" polar plot, the one that looks like an upside-down heart in Figure 8–6. Compared to its sensitivity to sounds coming straight from the front, this microphone is actually 30 dB less sensitive to sounds coming straight from the rear (180°)! If all the numbers (in decibels) were added together for all 360 degrees, and then divided by 360, an average 4.8-dB value would be found. This would be compared to the microphone's maximum sensitivity, namely to sounds coming from 0°. The hyper-cardioid polar plot has a slightly better average DI (some 6 dB) than the super-cardioid polar plot, which has an average DI of about 5.8 dB. In turn, the super-cardioid polar plot has a

Polar Plots for Directional Microphones

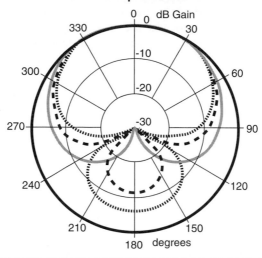

FIGURE 8–6 Idealized polar plots are shown for the omni-directional (the widest, outside circle) and also for various types of directional microphones. The round polar plot is that of the omni-directional microphone. It shows that the omni-directional microphone is equally sensitive to sounds originating from at directions (360°). The DI for this polar plot is 0, because the omni-directional microphone is no more sensitive to frontal sounds that it is to sounds coming from other directions. The light gray solid line shows a cardioid polar plot that looks like an upside-down heart. The dashed line polar plot with the smallest rear lobe is from the "super-cardioid" directional microphone. The remaining dotted line polar plot is known as "hyper-cardioid." According to Preves (1997), the cardioid microphone has a DI of 4.8 dB, the supercardioid directional microphone has a DI of 5.7 dB, and the hypercardioid directional microphone has a DI of 6.0 dB. Of course, DIs also depend on other factors, such as frequency.

slight better DI than the cardioid polar plot, with its DI of about 4.7dB (Dittberner, 2003). Most typical directional microphones for today's hearing aids show a DI of about 5 dB to 6dB. This means they are generally about 5 dB to 6 dB more sensitive to sounds directly from the front than they are to sounds coming from all other directions.

The polar plots shown in Figure 8–6 do not show frequency, and it is important to acknowledge that the DI varies for different frequencies, because speech (the main signal of interest) is comprised of many different frequencies. Furthermore, the clues or cues for recognizing speech are found more at some frequencies than at others. Therefore, a different weighting can be given for some frequencies than for others. This is known as the articulation index (AI), shown in Figure 8-7. This figure shows an audiogram with 100 dots, which represent the acoustic energy of speech. Each dot represents 1% of the speech

Articulation Index

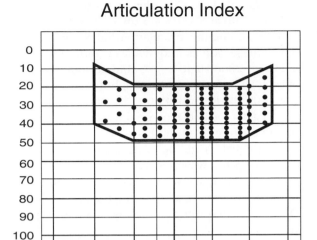

FIGURE 8–7   Unaided conversational level speech is plotted across the typical audiogram. The dots below one's hearing thresholds represent the speech that would be audible to the person; the dots above one's hearing thresholds represent the speech that is not audible. Note that there are exactly 100 dots with the range of unaided speech. Each dot represents 1% of the audible cues required in order to *understand* what was said. The count-the-dot audiogram can be used as a way to assign weight or importance to frequency regions of speech. Most of the dot density occurs between 1000 and 4000 Hz, especially around 2000 Hz. This means most speech cues required for the understanding of speech are found at these frequencies. According to this, polar plots and their respective DIs should be given different weights of importance. For example, a DI of 5 dB at 500 Hz would not be worth quite as much as a similar DI at 2000 Hz. Note. From An Easy Method For Calculating the Articulation Index, (Figure 1, p. 15), *The Hearing Journal, 43*(9), by Mueller, H. G., & Killion, M. C. (1990).

cues required for optimal speech recognition (Mueller & Killion, 1990). It is not surprising that the frequencies between 1000 and 4000 Hz have the most dots and are, therefore, given the most weight.

The benefit of directional microphone for speech intelligibility can, thus, be demonstrated through the use of the articulation index-based directivity index (AI-DI). The AI-DI results in a single number in decibels whereby to measure the overall effectiveness of a directional microphone (Roberts & Schulein, 1997; Killion, et al., 1998). It shows in decibels, the SNR improvement for listening to speech that would result if the background noise were turned down by that amount (ER-44 D-MIC data sheet, 1997). The AI-DI for a particular directional microphone is typically between 0 dB and 6 dB.

Let's look at an example here. Consider a fictitious directional microphone that provides a DI of 5.5 dB at 500 Hz, 4.5 dB at 1000 Hz, 4 dB at 2000 Hz, and 3.5 dB at 4000 Hz. According the articulation index shown in Figure 8–7, the weighting at each of these various frequencies is different: at 500 Hz it is 20%, at 1000 Hz it is 23%, at 2000 Hz it is 33%, and at 4000 Hz it is 24%. A simple multiplication of each DI by its particular weighting percentage yields 1.1 dB at 500 Hz, 1.04 dB at 1000 Hz, 1.32 dB at 2000 Hz, and .84 dB at 4000 Hz. Add up these values, and you get a total AI-DI of 4.3 dB.

Now, try the same exercise again; this time, however, multiply the DI for each frequency by an equal weighting of 25%, and then add up the weighted results. When you add up the weighted values, you'll arrive at a total AI-DI of 4.375 dB. "A man on a flying horse won't recognize the difference," so instead, look at the big picture; don't place all that much emphasis on the necessity or weighting the DIs at each frequency separately, when a simple average should give the basic idea.

Here's the "dirt" on directional microphone benefit. To correctly recognize 50% of speech, normal-hearing people require the speech to be at least as loud as the background noise (Killion, 1997a & b). Of course, the actual SNRs required for 50% performance may differ from lab to lab, depending on the acoustic properties of the speech signal and the types of noise used. For the sake of a simple explanation, however, let's say that for normal-hearing people to perform on some speech listening task, the speech had to be the same intensity as the background noise (0 dB SNR).

A loss of cochlear hair cells, resulting in a mild-moderate SNHL, necessitates an *additional* 5 dB in the level of speech relative to the noise, for the person to recognize 50% of it (Killion, 1997a & b). More pronounced degrees of SNHL naturally require even more SNR to perform at a similar speech recognition level. This is why manufacturers began to utilize directional microphone systems that could hit that magic number; a DI of 5 dB!

Killion's main message (1997a & b) was that directional microphones increase the SNR for speech sounds coming from the front by only a few (2 to 6) dB; although this may not sound like much, it really is, when the following is considered: *Every 1 dB of speech increase relative to the background noise results in a 10% improvement of speech recognition in noise!*

Subsequent measures have not shown this claim to be consistently obtained in difficult listening situations encountered in real life (Walden, Surr, & Cord, 2003). Measurement of directional effectiveness usually shows better results in laboratory testing situations than it does in the tougher listening situations presented by everyday surroundings. This is because in most laboratory testing environments (such as sound-treated booths), speech is typically presented at a 0° azimuth and noise is presented from speakers placed in other directions. Walden, et al., (2003) also caution against placing the noise-producing loudspeakers in the "nulls" of the polar plot. The nulls are the large indents in the polar plots (Figure 8–6) where the microphone's sensitivity reduction is the largest. Maximal directional benefit is generally achieved when the signal (speech) source is in front of and fairly close to the listener and when the noise source is coming from a distinctly different direction.

According to Ricketts (2003), factors that can create variability in predicted performance improvement are as follows. Microphones that have good directionality over a broad frequency range tend to provide more benefit than those that do not. Directionality in BTEs is generally similar to directionality in ITEs. Furthermore, the vent size also plays a part; the larger the vent, the poorer the DI. This occurs because the lows can escape out from the ear canal without being reduced in intensity by the directional microphone. Vent effects on DI values thus have an impact for the fitting of the up-and-coming open-ear BTEs, mentioned in Chapter 3.

All in all, however, directionality does provide an objective increase in speech reception performance in noise. Even when we cut Killion's optimistic (1997a & b) directional microphone benefit in half, a directional 5 dB increase in speech that results in 25% speech reception performance improvement is not too shabby.

The Present and Future for Directional Microphones

"*Adaptive directionality*" has also hit the marketplace (Dittberner, 2003). It is a feature commonly encountered on today's high-end digital hearing aids, where digital algorithms make changes and adjustments to the directionality depending on internal decision criteria. Adaptive directionality enables several things; for one, automatic selection of omni-directionality and directionality, depending on the listening environment. Clients can often choose between manual and automatic selection between these two modes. Adaptive directionality further enables an automatic selection among various available directional polar plots; again, this would depend on the specific listening environment. For example, if the noise source was determined to be directly behind the listener, a cardioid polar plot (as shown in Figure 8–6) would most likely be selected by the adaptive directionality. Other polar plots (super-cardioid, hyper-cardioid, and bi-directional), however, would automatically be selected if the listening situation called for these. In some digital hearing aids, the adaptive directionality automatically swings the polar plot so that its nulls (see Figure 8–6) face the noise source as much as possible.

Adaptive directionality typically uses the more expensive, quieter directional microphone system that consists of two omni-directional microphones placed side-by-side (dual-microphone processing described earlier in the chapter). Recall that unlike simple directional microphones, which rely on a critical (about 10 mm) physical distance between their two sound input ports, the more advanced dual-microphone directional systems rely on electronically produced time delays between the sounds arriving at each of the two ports. For these higher-end directional microphones, adaptive directionality provided by algorithms of the digital hearing aid enables optimal and automatic phase and frequency matching between the two omni-directional microphones. This prevents microphone "drift," which can degrade the once-achieved polar plots, and thus, maintains optimal directionality (Thompson, 2003). It really remains to be seen as to whether these adaptive directional systems truly result in improved speech-in-noise performance (Walden, et al., 2003).

A notable new development has very recently taken place in adaptive directionality, and that is the Directional Focus™, on the Innova™ product by Sonic Innovations. In addition to the features just mentioned, Directional Focus™ locates the direction of the competing noise, based on the phase differences of the two microphones, and then decreases the gain for these sounds! Thus, in addition to the microphone's decreased sensitivity to sounds that do not come from in front of the listener, there is also a deliberate gain reduction on the part of the amplifier itself. The amount of gain reduction (up to 6 dB) depends on the direction of the competing noise. In general, more attenuation is applied as the sound locates from the sides towards the rear. Directional Focus™ is actually a digital algorithm that is *completely separate* from the DNR algorithm provided by Sonic Innovations (more will be covered on this later in the chapter.) As such, it could theoretically be utilized on "lower-end" hearing aid products, which might not incorporate the Sonic Innovations DNR algorithm.

Together with their regular directional microphones, the AI-DIs provided with the addition of Directional Focus™, would bring astoundingly high numbers, into the double digits. New ANSI S3.22 standards of 2003 (Frye, 2005), however, prevent the usage of any adaptive algorithm while establishing DIs. As such, this adaptive feature of Directional Focus™ must be turned off while testing the directionality of the new Innova™ hearing aid. In the final analysis, however, it will be the clients who try this new form of adaptive directionality, who will tell us all how well it works in noise.

As mentioned earlier, second- and third-order directional systems are becoming more popular. The term "array microphones" is often used when discussing these directional microphone systems (Dittberner, 2003). Array microphones hold the promise of "beam forming." This is presently becoming an additional feature in high-end directional microphones. Beam forming is a directional microphone array with three or more ports! Beam forming, enabled by second- and third-order directional microphones, can increase the DI of a directional microphone system by making it even more directional, more tightly focused on frontal incoming sounds. In other words, beam forming makes a microphone system act like a magnifying glass for sound, or like a tunnel of directionality. Think about a hearing aid that could communicate via FM with a remote, pen-like beam forming device; the listener could engage in a conversation while sitting on a table in a noisy room, and turn the pen in the direction he/she wishes to hear. With beam forming, by far the loudest voice heard will be that person to whom the pen is pointing. Come to think of it, an FM system itself is like a "super-duper" directional microphone too; it acts to "bring the hearing aid up to the lips of the speaker," thus increasing the SNR!

Examples of beam forming are already available. The Siemens Triano™ was the first digital BTE to utilize three microphone ports. Two other examples that come to mind are Phonak's Microzoom™ and the Lexis™, available from Oticon, Bernafon, and Starkey. Each of these systems consists of a "boot" fit to the BTE, and a directional microphone array consisting of at least three sound entry ports. The microphone can be worn around the speaker's neck, like an FM system transmitter, or else it can be placed on a table top near the listener and pointed in the direction from which the listener wishes to hear. The transmitter can be adjusted to provide a beam forming focus on incoming sound from a specific direction. This sound is then sent via FM radio waves to the boot fastened to the listener's BTE. These products increase the DI up to about 7 dB or 8 dB.

Directional microphones are basically understood as a way to increase the SNR for those with hearing loss. They can be construed as a way to work *around* the problem of damaged cochlear hair cells. It is presently impossible to work *through* the problem; we cannot repair the damaged cochlea, nor can we truly subtract noise from target speech by digital technology (more is discussed on this in the next section). We can, however, deliberately make speech more intense than the background noise so that the client can more easily separate them. This is what a directional microphone does. To give a geographical analogy, directional microphones can be considered a way of avoiding the necessity of boating over the treacherous Niagara Falls; they provide a parallel (Welland) canal, to sail around the obstacle.

DIGITAL NOISE REDUCTION

The removal of background noise from speech is often been touted as the main virtue of digital hearing aids. Clients commonly come into the clinic waving newspaper ads that mention noise reduction. Compared to directional microphones, DNR is a lot newer and more expensive way to deal with background noise. It is also very poorly explained and understood by the public. Everyone wants it; let's face it, the three main complaints about hearing aids are: background noise, feedback, and occlusion effect. Removal of background noise from speech has often been touted as a promising virtue of digital hearing aids. Only digital hearing aids provide this feature. One more thing: Schum (2003) points out that hearing aids have not been the first to use noise reduction. The military and also the telecommunications industry have been using it too.

For the sake of complete honesty, it must be stressed that an actual sampling and consequent removal or *subtraction* of background noise from speech is beyond what any digital hearing aid can presently deliver. This is especially true if the background noise is not stationary, such as the babble of background speech. Digital hearing aids with a few channels can indeed sample stationary noise as being distinct from speech, but to separate and subtract fluctuating background noise would require many more channels than most digital hearing aids now employ. As mentioned in Chapter 3, speech is a rapidly fluctuating signal that varies constantly in amplitude, frequency, and time. To subtract background noise from speech would require many more than the number of channels commonly used in hearing aids today, because the frequency regions where the speech and noise "collide" might be very narrow. A much "finer-toothed comb" than is now feasible with today's DSP capabilities would be necessary to achieve this fine an extraction. Furthermore, a sampling of speech and a sampling of noise would need to be employed at a high rate of units per second. Any noise that is sampled between the stops and starts of speech syllables could be extracted, but such a noise subtraction might at the same time also unintentionally remove some of the most important cues for distinguishing and categorizing elements of the target speech. The necessary DSP calculating power and speed to sample background speech babble from target speech cannot yet be readily housed in a small computer chip that would fit inside (or behind) someone's ear canal.

Present digital technology does offer a more plausible solution to the problem of speech in background noise: namely, noise *reduction, or attenuation.* This can be accomplished more readily with DSP than with analog circuits, because digital hearing aids can actively reduce the gain in channels where the background noise is most present. In any one channel then, the DNR algorithm will reduce the gain for both the speech and the noise (the baby does indeed get thrown out with the bathwater)! This certainly will *not provide an objective improvement* for speech recognition in noise (as can be provided with directional microphones), but it will accomplish something else; it can *enhance the client's listening subjective comfort* in noise.

Clinical Benefits of DNR

In Chapter 7, we looked at how digital noise reduction basically works. Here, we will examine its clinical benefits. In this way, one can better appreciate how it compares and complements the use of directional microphones. The heart of DNR is in the right place. The main problem is that noise removal from speech is easier said than done. Speech and noise are inextricably mixed together. Digital noise reduction may remove noise, but then at the same time, it also tends to remove speech cues too. Instead of touting how much speech reception can be *improved* by DNR, manufacturers would be better off describing and promoting how *little* their noise reduction algorithms might *damage, or otherwise reduce* speech understanding. Again, the emPHAsis should be placed on a different syLLAble.

Here's why: A retrospective look *way* back into your studies might help highlight the wonders of speech perception and at the same time, the inadequacies of present-day DNR. Figure 8–8 shows a spectrographic analysis of three speech syllables: ba, da, and ga. We make "ba" by putting our two lips together, we make "da" by putting the tip of our tongues against the bumpy ridge behind our front teeth, and we make "ga" by squeezing the back of our tongues against the roof of our mouths. The horizontal axis shows time, the vertical axis shows frequency, and the thick bands show the resonances, or formants, of the vocal tract while saying these syllables. Note that the lowest resonance or formant is identical for each of the three syllables. Note also, the even the little, tiny points at the ends of the bottom formants are identical. These points are the transitions, small, but all-important speech cues that help us determine the differences among similar-sounding speech syllables.

Now take a look at the second, or higher-frequency formants. These are also similar in frequency across the syllables. It is only the tiny transitions of the

Critical Speech Cues
on Spectrogram

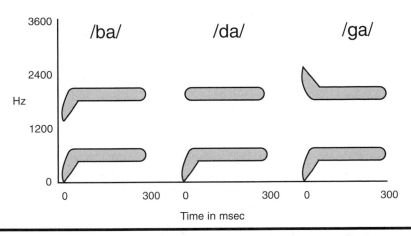

FIGURE 8–8   A spectrogram shows all three dimensions of sound: frequency, intensity, and time. The thick bars in the figure are the resonances of the vocal tract (formants), as produced when uttering the three syllables /ba/, /da/, and /ga/. Note that the two resonances shown for each of the three syllables occur at the same frequencies. The only acoustic property that makes them distinct from each other are the small tails (formant transitions) that occur for the second or higher resonances of /ba/ and /ga/. For any one syllable (e.g., /ba/), progressive, tiny changes to this transition does not produce the perception of a different syllable (e.g., /da/) until the changes pass a certain point of magnitude. Past that point, only the other syllable (e.g., /da/) will be heard. In other words, we do not hear the tiny progressive changes, because we do not normally produce these tiny changes. We either say /ba/ or /da/.

higher-frequency formants that make up the acoustic differences among the three syllables shown here. If we want to make "ba" sound more like "da," we'd have to cut off some of its second formant transition. Let's do it really gradually; take off just the very tip of the higher-formant transition for the syllable "ba." If we now played these two formants, we'd still hear "ba." If we took off a tiny bit more and played the two formants, we'd still hear "ba." If we took of a *little* bit more, we'd still hear "ba." If we took off a tiny little bit more, we'd now hear "da."

The motor theory of speech perception (Denes & Pinson, 1993) states that the reason we cannot hear the transition sounds between "ba" and "da" is because we cannot physically utter them. More specifically, we cannot physically *make* a speech motion that is half way between the productions of "ba" and "da." It's called "categorical perception." If we think we hear something in the middle, we immediately lump it into one or another category. Perhaps a dog or cat could hear the transitions in between "ba" and "da," but we who talk and *say* these syllables cannot. Think of how a Japanese person may have difficulty discerning between "r" and "l"; this would again be because he/she does not normally produce and distinguish between these sounds in that language.

At any rate, the purpose here is not to discuss speech perception per se. It is, however, very important to appreciate how a DNR algorithm might easily throw these tiny, but all-important acoustic transitions out with the bath water when reducing background noise.

Figure 8–9 shows another way of looking at the same thing. Both panels show an odd assortment of tiny vertical points. Actually, they give a visual idea as to the energy of a sentence spoken at a conversational speech level. The vertical axis is time, the horizontal axis is frequency, and the height of the points show intensity. The low frequencies of speech (the tall spikes on the left side of each panel) have the most energy, while the high frequencies of speech (the low points on the right of each panel) have the least energy. With some imagination, the series of points actually look a bit like mountain ranges with trees, descending towards the sea. The left panel shows the speech sample spoken in quiet. The right panel shows the same speech sample with background noise present. Again, imagine a flood filling the low-lying plains and valleys. One must ask how a digital "claw" would be expected to enter the picture and remove all of the noise without at the same time, damaging the trees. This scenario can be taken as a visual analogy of the difficulties and challenges encountered by DNR.

The algorithm for DNR is really an example of artificial intelligence. DNR basically works by analyzing the nature of the sound coming into the hearing aid. It samples the incoming sound and determines whether the sample fits into the category of noise or the category of speech. As mentioned before in Chapter 7, if it is determined to be noise, then the hearing aid temporarily reduces the gain in any channel where it was sensed, by some 5 dB to 20 dB.

Why Are There No Single-Channel Digital Hearing Aids Offering DNR?

Has anyone ever wondered why single-channel digital hearing aids are not normally available? Perhaps this is because digital hearing aid technology is considered to be beyond that of the high-end multi-channel analog technology, so it would be pointless to go back in time. But there could also be another reason. Bearing in mind what we have discussed so far regarding DNR, think about how DNR would work in a one-channel digital hearing aid. Figure 8–10 shows a fictitious single-channel digital hearing aid, with a broad gain frequency response that is amplifying the sounds of incoming speech. The speech sounds differ in intensity (as we saw in Chapter 2), but for the purposes of illustration here, the gain is fairly flat across all frequencies.

Now imagine that background noise has come into the picture, and the DNR algorithm kicks in. The gain over the entire frequency response is simply reduced by some 5 dB to 20 dB. This amounts to a simple gain reduction; one could simply have turned down the volume control! This is not truly going to increase the reception and understanding of speech in the background noise.

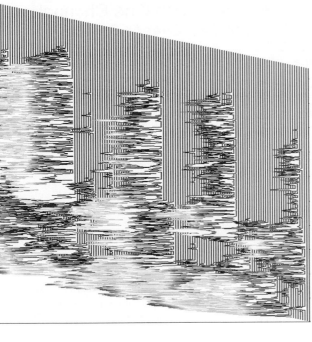

Speech in Quiet   **Speech in Noise**

Frequency   Frequency

Time

FIGURE 8–9 For both panels, the vertical axis represents time, and the horizontal axis represents frequency. In human speech, the most intense sounds produced are the low-frequency vowels and voiced consonants. In comparison, the unvoiced consonants are relatively higher in frequency and softer in intensity. The spikes seen on the left are thus taller, and the spikes seen on the right are much shorter. Speech in quiet is shown in the left panel. Speech in noise is shown in the right panel. The noise is the depicted as the black horizontal lines that cover up the lower spikes (softer speech sounds).

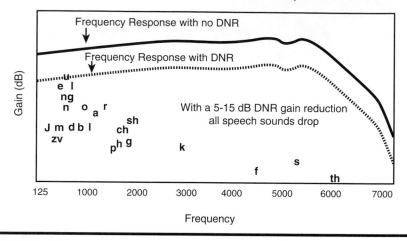

FIGURE 8–10   DNR is not typically offered in single-channel digital hearing aids because this would only amount to an overall reduction of gain across the entire frequency range of the hearing aid. This would be akin to simply reducing the VC.

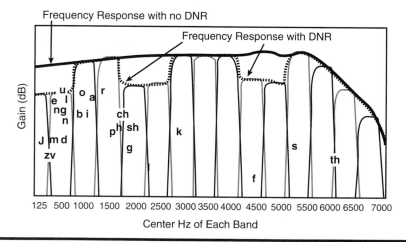

FIGURE 8–11   DNR is most effective when used in each of many frequency bands of a digital hearing aid. With many frequency bands, the width of each band is relatively narrow. If noise is sensed in any one band, the gain is accordingly reduced. This results in less overall gain reduction than would take place in a single-channel digital hearing aid.

Now, consider a fictitious, many-channel digital hearing aid, shown in Figure 8–11. Consider also that the DNR algorithm works separately and independently in each and every channel. Imagine that noise has once again come into the picture. In this digital hearing aid, the DNR is working over very narrow frequency bands. The result is *less* unnecessary reduction of gain, with *less* negative impact upon the aided speech signal. Still, however, we would be hard pressed to say that speech reception has *objectively* improved. The best way to surmise the effects of noise reduction in a many-channel digital hearing aid is to say that it damages or ruins the aided speech signal to a lesser degree than the same thing would do in a one-channel digital hearing aid. Think about DNR like buying a car as an investment; it's not a matter of whether you lose money on it or not, but the question is rather more like how fast you will lose the money.

To the author's knowledge, Sonic Innovations remains the only manufacturer of digital hearing aids that has produced an objective, albeit *slight* improvement in speech reception in speech-weighted steady-state, background noise (Bray & Nilsson, 2000; Mueller & Ricketts, 2003). For the most part, however, ReSound, a prominent hearing aid manufacturer, once said it best in advertisements of their DNR: The challenge for optimal speech reception in noise is to ". . . minimize the impact upon speech."

DIRECTIONAL MICROPHONES AND DNR AS A TEAM

Conventional wisdom is that directional microphones *objectively* improve speech recognition in background noise, while DNR *subjectively* enhances listening comfort in background noise. One could think of directional microphones as the head (or the science) and of DNR as the heart (or the art). Together, they could be construed as working well as a team (Venema, 1999).

Of the two, however, DNR is by far the more expensive option. To that end, it is most interesting (and disconcerting) that directional microphones are more commonly found on higher-cost hearing aids. While studying many hearing aid features and their respective costs, Punch (2001) consistently found a strong association between directional microphones and high-end hearing aids. According to Kochkin (1993), problems in background noise are a big reason why people stow their hearing aids away in drawers. At a large American Academy Convention featured session in 2001(Laurel Christensen, Todd Ricketts, Victor Bray, Wouter Dreschler, and the author gave presentations on the features and clinical benefits of directional microphones versus digital noise reduction), the author recalls Kochkin asking the question as to why manufacturers consistently seem to save directional microphones for their more expensive, high-end hearing aids. I had to agree with his point. Perhaps it is time for directional microphones to be routinely included as a standard feature on all hearing aids that can possibly house them!

Compared to digital noise reduction, directional microphones can be a relatively simple solution to the problem of background noise. What's more, they can be featured in low-end hearing aids (Venema, 2001). As discussed earlier in this chapter, the clinical benefits of directionality have been repeatedly shown. Any device that increases the intensity of speech compared to background noise (directionality) can provide huge benefits for the end user.

It is obvious that digital hearing aids have come and are here to stay. Furthermore, no one needs to persuade most clinicians that high-end digital hearing aids can include lots of extra features and benefits. But for the millions of consumers who are unable or unwilling to pay the several thousands dollars that today's digital hearing aids cost, the inclusion of simple directional microphones on low-end digital hearing aids could spell a wonderful success for our industry. It would demonstrate to clinicians that hearing aid manufacturers are truly thinking about the trends that are taking place right now. Making directionality a standard feature of low-end analog hearing aids would also be a good way to enhance and promote less-expensive digital products.

If manufacturers ever took this step, it is to be hoped that they will be vocal about it, by boldly advertising directionality as a low-cost alternative to more advanced technology. In doing this, they just might surprise their customers and consumers with their common sense. Perhaps directionality should be a standard feature on every hearing aid that can include it, not just an option. If manufacturers and hearing health care professionals want to reduce returns for credit and also reach a much greater segment of the hearing-impaired population, it behooves us to provide directional microphones on low-end, single-channel, analog hearing aids. Recent advances in technology have increased the complexity of hearing aids, sometimes to the point of being overwhelming. Some effective simplicity would be a breath of fresh air.

SUMMARY

- Directional microphones are an older technology that has continually evolved to where it is today. Directional microphones are most sensitive to frontal sounds and less sensitive to sounds coming from other directions.

- Directional microphones tend to increase the SNR, providing that the signal (speech) comes from the front, and the noise comes from other directions. This is why they often provide objective improvement for understanding speech in background noise.

- Digital hearing aids change sound into numerical or digital information. These digits can be manipulated at will, by long sets of commands, called "algorithms." The fact that digits can be manipulated in almost any conceivable way is what makes DSP hearing aids more flexible and adaptive to different listening environments than their analog counterparts.

- Digital hearing aids typically are programmable and multi-channel. They often have many more than two channels. They combine many forms of static and dynamic compression. They also provide expansion and DNR.

- DNR is known to enhance subjective listening comfort in noisy environments. Listeners do not have to adjust the VC as much.

- Directional microphones, with their objective SNR improvements, can be considered the science or the head. DNR, with its subjective comfort enhancements, can be considered the art or the heart. Together, on digital hearing aids, they work well as a team.

REVIEW QUESTIONS

1. According to the approach of this text, hearing aids should do two things:
   a. improve speech reception and enhance listening comfort in noise.
   b. increase audibility and increase the signal-to-noise ratio (SNR).
   c. increase choice of hearing aid selection and lower cost.
   d. amplify the traveling wave and sharpen it.

2. Directional microphones were first invented:
   a. in 1998, right after DNR appeared on the scene.
   b. in the 1960s.
   c. by the military, some 50 years ago.
   d. none of the above

3. Directional microphones:
   a. enhance subjective listening comfort in noise.
   b. objectively increase SNR.
   c. help the listener locate the direction of sound.
   d. can only be found on digital hearing aids.

4. Directional microphones generally work poorest when the speech and noise:
   a. are of equal intensity.
   b. come from opposite directions.
   c. come from the same direction.
   d. all of the above

5. A general resurgence in directional microphone popularity occurred in:
   a. 1998, right after DNR appeared on the scene.
   b. the 1960s.

    c. the 1980s.

    d. by the military, some 50 years ago.

6. A directional polar plot by itself has one thing missing; namely,

    a. intensity.

    b. phase.

    c. frequency.

    d. decibels.

7. The most important audible frequency cue for understanding speech is:

    a. 500 Hz.

    b. 1000 Hz.

    c. 2000 Hz.

    d. 4000 Hz.

8. DNR is known to:

    a. enhance subjective listening comfort in noise.

    b. objectively increase SNR.

    c. help the listener locate the direction of speech.

    d. be found on single-channel digital hearing aids.

9. DNR is generally:

    a. a low-cost option found in digital hearing aids.

    b. a higher-cost feature than directional microphones.

    c. an effective way to remove noise from speech.

    d. an effective way to increase the SNR.

10. According to Kochkin (1993), the biggest single reason people reject the hearing aids is:

    a. excessive background noise.

    b. too much occlusion effect.

    c. excessive feedback.

    d. none of the above

RECOMMENDED READINGS

Mueller, G., & Ricketts, T. (2005). Digital noise reduction: Much ado about nothing? *The Hearing Journal, 58*(1): 10–17.

Walden, B., Surr, R., & Cord, M. (2003). Real-world performance of directional microphones hearing aids. *The Hearing Journal, 56*(11): 40–47.

REFERENCES

Bray, V., & Nilsson, M. (2000). Objective test results support benefits of a DSP noise reduction system. *The Hearing Review,* 7(11): 60-65.

Bray, V., & Nilsson, M. (2001). Additive SNR benefits of signal processing features in a directional hearing aid. *The Hearing Review,* 8(12): 48-51, 62.

Denes, P., & Pinson, E. (1993). *The speech chain* (2nd ed). New York: W. H. Freeman and Company.

Dittberner, A. (2003). What's new in directional-microphone systems? How does it help the user? *The Hearing Journal,* 56(4): 10-18.

ER-44 D-MIC data sheet. (1997). Etymotic Research, 61 Martin Lane, Elk Grove Village, IL 60007.

Frye, G. (2005). Understanding the ANSI standard as a tool for assessing hearing instrument functionality. *The Hearing Review,* 12(5): 22-27.

Killion, M. C., (1997a). "I can hear what people say, but I can't understand them." *The Hearing Review,* 4(12): 8-14.

Killion, M. C. (1997b). The SIN report: Circuits haven't solved the hearing-in-noise problem. *The Hearing Journal,* 50(10): 28-34.

Killion, M. C., Schulein, R., Christensen, L., Fabry, D., Revit, L., Niquette, P., & Chung, K. (1998). Real-world performance of an ITE directional micro-phone. *The Hearing Journal,* 51(4): 24-38.

Kochkin, S. (1993). MarkeTrac III identifies key factors in customer satisfaction. *The Hearing Journal,* 46(4): 36-37.

Kochkin, S. (2001). Personal communication.

Kuk, F. K., (1996). Real-world consumer satisfaction with a user-controlled, multi-microphone communication system. *Hearing Instruments,* 47(1): 24-28.

Levitt, H. (2001). Noise reduction in hearing aids: a review. *Journal of Rehabilitation Research and Development,* 38(1): 111-121.

Mueller, H., & Killion, M. C. (1990). An easy method for calculating the articulation index. *The Hearing Journal,* 43(9): 14-17.

Mueller H., & Ricketts, T. (2000). Directional-microphone hearing aids: An up-date. *The Hearing Journal,* 53(5): 10-19.

Mueller, G., & Ricketts, T. (2005). Digital noise reduction: Much ado about noth-ing? *The Hearing Journal,* 58(1): 10-17.

Preves, D. (1997, July). Directional microphone use in ITE hearing instruments. *The Hearing Review,* 4(7): 21-27.

Punch, J. (2001). Technologic and functional features of hearing aids: What are their relative costs? *The Hearing Journal,* 54(6): 32-44.

Ricketts, T. (2003). How fitting, patient, and environmental factors affect direc-tional benefit. *The Hearing Journal,* 56(11): 31-39.

Roberts, M., & Schulein, R. (1997). *Etymotic research. Objective measurement of the intelligibility performance of hearing aids.* Based on paper presented at the 103rd Convention at the Audio Engineering Society in New York City, September 26–29, 1997.

Schum, D. (2003). Noise reduction via signal processing: (1) Strategies used in other industries. *The Hearing Journal, 56*(5): 27–32.

Thompson, S. (2003). Tutorial on microphone technologies for directional hearing aids. *The Hearing Journal, 56*(11): 14–21.

Venema, T. (1999). Three ways to fight noise: Directional microphones, DSP algorithms, and expansion. *The Hearing Journal, 52*(10): 58–62.

Venema, T. (2001). Directional microphones for low-end hearing aids. *The Hearing Journal, 54*(10): 48

Walden, B., Surr, R., & Cord, M. (2003). Real-world performance of directional microphone hearing aids. *The Hearing Journal, 56*(11): 40–47.

Classes of Hearing Aid Amplifiers, A, B, D, and H: Where's Class C?

Digital hearing aids today normally use the class D amplifier; furthermore, the class D amplifier no longer houses both the amplifier and receiver as was the case in yesterday's analog hearing aids. More is mentioned about class D amplifiers further below. What follows is a general, course description of amplifer classes, just for the reader's information.

In analog (nondigital) hearing aids, the most basic way to categorize amplifiers is to break them down into the way in which they amplify or provide gain. The amplifier class is the fundamental block on which the rest of the hearing aid characteristics are built. That a hearing aid provides linear gain or compression is independent of the amplifier class. At the root of any linear or compression hearing aid circuit is the class to which its amplifier belongs.

Each type, or class, of hearing aid amplifier can be either linear or compression. For example, spec sheets from many hearing aid manufacturers used to show hearing aids available in class A linear, class A compression, class D linear, class D compression, class D WDRC, and so on. WDRC was usually associated with class D, and the K Amp^{TM}, as a WDRC circuit, was also built on a class D amplifier/receiver.

Class A amplifiers are the oldest analog amplifier type. They are also the least expensive. As long as the gain requirements are moderate, the class A amplifier produces low distortion (Longwell & Gawinski, 1992). The main problem with class A amplifiers is that they constantly use battery power whether they are amplifying an input sound or not. Class A amplifiers are, thus, not the most efficient hearing aid amplifiers.

The reason class A amplifiers constantly use up battery power is that a bias current is necessary from the battery to keep the diaphragm of the receiver at a middle position. The receiver of the hearing aid is the part that receives sound from the parts of the circuit that precede it and sends the sound out into the ear canal of the listener. The diaphragm of the receiver wobbles back and forth and in so doing it transduces or changes the electrical energy of the circuit back into sound for the listener. The diaphragm has to be kept at a middle position so it can vibrate freely on both sides of the middle position. The power required to do this usurps power from the battery for the whole time the hearing aid is turned on. If the diaphragm is not kept at a middle position as it vibrates, it hits the sides of the receiver wall, resulting in peak clipping and distortion.

Class B amplifiers are like two class A amplifiers stuck together, back to back. As a result, they are often larger than class A amplifiers. Each of the two active parts of a Class B amplifier works on opposite sides of the alternating sound signal. Due to the equal and opposite actions of the class B amplifier, the diaphragm of the receiver rests at a center position. No bias current is necessary. Class B amplifiers can provide more gain and output than a class A, because the full battery voltage of the hearing aid is applied to each sideways swing of the diaphragm's movement. The diaphragm can thus move in a larger side-to-side motion. This is why class B amplifiers are often referred to as "push/pull" amplifiers and why they are associated with high-power hearing aids.

Because a bias current is not needed to keep the diaphragm centered, the class B amplifier is more efficient in battery consumption than the class A amplifier. When there is no sound coming into the hearing aid, the class B amplifier does not use up much power. The battery consumption increases only as the signal going through the amplifier increases.

Class C stands for a class of very efficient amplifiers found in high-frequency radio transmitters. This type of amplifier is not at all appropriate for hearing aid circuits, so it is not used. Class C does not stand for compression.

In analog hearing aids, the class D amplifier is unique in that it is integrated into the receiver of the hearing aid. Actually, the class D amplifier is a small class A amplifier housed along with a pulse width modulator inside the receiver of the hearing aid. A high-frequency pulse is mixed along with the incoming sound signal and the result is a modulated pulse. This modulated pulse controls the opening and closing of four switches, which in turn control the current that goes through the receiver. Two of the switches allow the positive part of the current to go through, and two of them allow the negative part of the current to go through. As mentioned at the outset, class D amplifiers are normally used in today's digital hearing aids.

Class D amplifiers are very efficient, which results in relatively low battery power consumption. Similar to the class B amplifier, no bias current is needed to keep the diaphragm of the receiver in a center position. In fact, some power is actually returned to the battery during class D amplifier operation. The full battery voltage of the class D amplifier is applied to each half of the alternating sideways swing of the diaphragm. This results in increased gain and output, which is also similar to class B amplifiers. Other benefits of class D amplifiers in hearing aids is decreased distortion and extended high-frequency emphasis. These can increase the quality of sound for the listener (Longwell & Gawinski, 1992).

The class H amplifier is a relative newcomer for hearing aids. It is actually a class A amplifier with some special added circuitry. The added circuitry adjusts the typical bias current of a class A amplifier, according to the intensity of the sound input. As the input sound is increased, the bias current (needed to keep the diaphragm in a middle position) is also increased. The class H amplifier is efficient because, like the class B and D amplifiers, its battery power consumption depends on the sound input level and the current the hearing aid really needs to do its job.

REFERENCE

Longwell, T. F., & Gawinski, M. J., (1992). Fitting strategies for the 90s: Class D amplification. *The Hearing Journal, 45*(0): 2-5.

APPENDIX B

Answers to Summary Questions

Chapter 1

1. b   2. c   3. a   4. d   5. a   6. d   7. c   8. b   9. c   10. d

Chapter 2

1. c   2. a   3. b   4. a   5. b   6. c   7. a   8. d   9. b   10. d

Chapter 3

1. b   2. a   3. d   4. b   5. a   6. b   7. b   8. a
9. c   10. d

Chapter 4

1. c   2. a   3. c   4. c   5. d   6. a   7. c   8. d
9. b   10. a

Chapter 5

1. a   2. a   3. c   4. d   5. b   6. a   7. a   8. c   9. a
10. b   11. c   12. b   13. c   14. 50 dB   15. 105 dB SPL
16. 45 dB   17. 70 dB   18. 141 dB SPL   19. 142 dB SPL   20. 35 dB

Chapter 6

1. d   2. d   3. d   4. c   5. b   6. b   7. b   8. b
9. a   10. d

Chapter 7

1. b   2. a   3. c   4. b   5. a   6. d   7. a   8. c
9. d   10. d

Chapter 8

1. b   2. c   3. b   4. c   5. a   6. c   7. c   8. a
9. b   10. a

Index